VAGUS NERVE:

THE ULTIMATE SELF HELP GUIDE FOR ANXIETY THERAPY THROUGH VAGUS NERVE TREATMENT.

Introduction

All cranial nerves are also classified with specific names that are based on Roman numerals. These names vary according to that particular cranial nerves' location within the brain. For example, the vagus nerve is also called 'cranial nerve X' as it is the tenth nerve in the system.

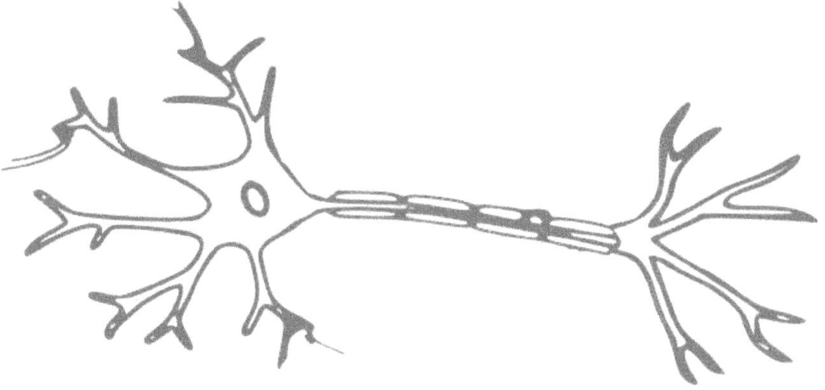

As the vagus nerve is so closely related to many other parts of the body and how they function, it can more often than not be used as a clear indicator of nerve damage when something else in the body begins to shut down or experience problems. Have you ever gone to the doctor and had them test your gag reflex? Say aaah!

This is often done with a cotton swab that they will then tickle the back and sides of your throat with, thus causing you to want to gag. When they do this, they are testing your vagus nerve, and so if you do not have a gag reflex when this not-so-fun part of your check up is happening, it may be an indicator that there is something wrong with your vagus nerve. This would then give the doctors somewhere to start with any treatments needing to be done, when they are looking for the root cause of your ailments. There is not a lot of point in treating symptoms if we can't get to the bottom of everything and fix the problem once and for all.

The vagus nerve is a large factor in the sensitivity of mucous membranes in the respiratory system and plays a massive role in transmitting the strength and rhythm of each breath you take as well as the frequency of your breaths. The vagus nerve also affects the larynx, esophagus, trachea, pharynx, as well as the bronchi, and will also assist with administering nerve fibers to the heart, pancreas, liver and last but not least, the stomach.

The vagus nerve will also have an almost reverse effect too, where not only is it delivering information from the brain to each of these organs, but it is also sending signals from the organs to go back to the brain to react accordingly. In order for this to happen, the vagus nerve contains two separate bunches of nerve cells that are connecting the organs and body to the brain stem.

These cells allow the brain to receive information from the organs relating to their different functions, and can therefore monitor what is happening within our bodies, should the need arise to fix something that has gone faulty.

The vagus nerve's main functions are large contributing factors toward the autonomic nervous system, which mainly consists of two parts, namely the parasympathetic and sympathetic parts. These two parts will be discussed in further detail later in our book under the autonomic nervous system.

So what exactly is it that this vagus nerve will affect, you may ask? Let's have a look:

- Sensory factors such as the throat, lungs, heart, and abdomen are affected.

- Special sensory factors include taste sensations behind your tongue.

- Your motor functions such as movement for the muscles in the neck that are directly responsible for speech as well as the swallowing motion.

- Your parasympathetic functions that are in charge of the entire gastro-intestinal tract, respiratory system, as well as the function of your heart rate.

Other effects from the vagus nerve include the following:

- Delivering information between the digestive system and the brain.

- Deep breathing in order to achieve a higher sense of relaxation, where the vagus nerve will communicate with the diaphragm allowing you to hold a larger breath.

- The vagus nerve will send out anti-inflammatory signals, allowing the body to naturally reduce any inflammation and swelling in the system.

- The vagus nerve can also be used to lower your blood pressure as well as your heart rate, as when the vagus nerve is in an overactive state, it can cause the heart to be unable to pump enough blood through your body which may also lead to organ damage.

- The vagus nerve is also responsible for dealing with stress, fear, and anxiety, which are also directly linked to your gut. This is where the saying "gut feeling" originated. The signals then sent through the vagus nerve will help a person to recover from a stressful or scary situation.

A few other magical moments that this powerful little tool can offer us when used correctly is that it can block the cortisol hormone in your system as well as other oxidizing agents that tend to deteriorate the brain and body and cause our systems to age faster than they should.

We can also confirm that this nerve can help us to overcome sleep disorders so that we may have a more restful night. Great news for any insomniacs out there! This also in turn can help reduce any chronic stress and tension headaches.

Overall this nerve can help us live a healthier, longer life once we have learnt how to use it to our advantage.

Where is the Vagus Nerve Located?

The vagus nerve comes from Latin meaning wandering nerve, which is aptly named due to it being the longest cranial nerve and reaching all the way down to the digestive system from the brain stem.

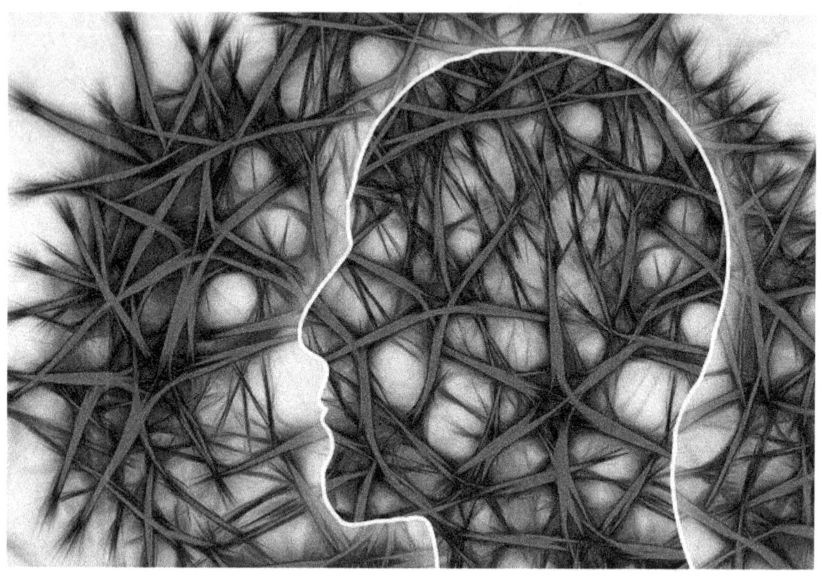

The sensory components of the vagus nerve are divided into two parts, namely somatic components which help with feeling sensations in your muscles or on your skin, and then visceral components which are sensations that are felt in your body's organs.

Technically, there are two vagus nerves, being the left and the right, but doctors will normally refer to the pair as one whole vagus nerve.

The vagus nerve is in the cranium, much like the spinal cord, and from there it moves down into the neck, passes through a number of organs, and ends up in the abdomen. The vagus nerve goes from the medulla oblongata and passes itself between the inferior cerebellar peduncle where it will then further extend through the jugular foramina and moves in a posterolateral form in between the internal carotid artery and the internal jugular vein along its route down the neck to the chest and abdomen.

This goes to show just how long the vagus nerve truly is, and even then, you find that it goes that extra step further in contributing towards the viscera where the colon lies.

If we split the pair up to have a look at each of the two vagus nerves separately on their way down the nervous system, you will find that the right vagus nerve allows the right recurrent laryngeal nerve to hook itself around the subclavian artery, and then passes up into the neck in between the esophagus and tracheal passage. The right vagus nerve will then cross over into the right subclavian artery itself, and then passes alongside behind the superior vena cava, and further goes down to the back of the right main bronchus. This nerve then contributes to pulmonary, cardiac, and esophageal jungle. It lastly becomes the posterior vagal trunk at the bottom and last end of the esophagus, and from there it will enter the diaphragm.

Next up is the left vagus nerve which then moves into the chest cavity between the left carotid artery and left subclavian artery. The left vagus nerve then allows the left recurrent laryngeal nerve to hook itself around the aortic arch, which ascends between the esophagus and trachea. The left vagus nerve further branches out into making up the jungle in the pulmonary system, then further enters into the abdomen as the anterior vagal trunk in the esophageal hiatus of the diaphragm.

Functions of the Vagus Nerve

One of the greatest anomalies about the vagus nerve is that it is the major parasympathetic nerve of the entire body! This nerve is supplying parasympathetic fibers throughout the nervous system to all the most important organs of the body, especially focusing on those within the abdomen, chest cavity, neck and head. The vagus nerve is in charge of many of the body's main functions that all seem a bit strange to be linked together. Have you noticed that when you clean your ears out and stimulate the ear canal, you cough? That is because the cough reflex is directly linked to ear canal stimulation.

The vagus nerve is also directly linked to your gag reflex when the back and sides of the throat are stimulated, it is linked to slowing your heart rate, and it can control your sweating and regulate your blood pressure. It can also stimulate peristalsis of the gastrointestinal tract as well as being able to control your vascular tone.

The vagus nerve has both sensory as well as motor functions that keep us ticking the way we should. Some of these functions include:

- The stimulation of muscles in the soft palate, which is in the roof of your mouth, as well as stimulating the larynx and pharynx inside your throat.

- Heart stimulation, which thereafter helps to lower your heart rate as well as regulate your blood pressure.

- The stimulation of the digestive tract in order to help you with digestion and passing your food through your system. This also includes stimulation of the esophagus.

- Stimulation of the sensitive skin behind your ears as a sensory piece, as well as sending information to the brain to trigger reflexes when stimulation is affecting the outer ear canal as well as the throat. You will also find that it plays a part in your taste sensations at the back of your mouth where the root of your tongue is.

When the vagus nerve gets stimulated very suddenly without any warning, you can cause a reaction called the vasovagal reflex to happen. When you get a vasovagal reflex, you often find that it causes a sudden drop in blood pressure as well as your heart rate will slow down dramatically.

There are some people who are unfortunately prone to getting these reflexes although it is most commonly found due to stress, high amounts of pain, getting a sudden fright or even from a gastrointestinal problem from something you may have eaten that didn't quite agree with your insides.

When this vasovagal reflex does happen, it will cause your heart rate and blood pressure to drop very quickly, most often causing loss of consciousness or fainting. This is a condition that is called vasovagal syncope.

When the vagus nerve gets stimulated for therapeutic effects, you will find that you are able to have complete control over your body!

You can stimulate the vagus nerve to stop a nasty hiccup episode that is relentless, and doctors will often use the vagus nerve to help them diagnose a potential heart murmur or to treat depression.

In order for your brain to know the current status of what is happening to the organs around your body, it needs the signals from the vagus nerve to bounce back through those organs and send a sort of 'report' back to the brain in order to react further.

The vagus nerve has become so important in the medical industry that doctors are now finding that they can stimulate the vagus nerve using a device that gets placed in your chest, somewhat like a pacemaker, and send signals to the nerve through this device in order to get certain reactions from your body. Vagus nerve blocking is also fast becoming a popular method of treatment, especially aiding in weight loss as it has become far more superior to that of gastric bypass surgery!

Let's go into some further details on the functions of the vagus nerve in medical cases.

The vagus nerve in relation to the heart is quite possibly the most important case of all. The right vagus nerve leads straight on to supply the sinus node, and can then cause sinus bradycardia when the right vagus nerve gets stimulated. The left vagus nerve leads on to the AV node which can then cut off stimulation to or block the heart when it gets stimulated. In blocking this particular receptor, you are then able to control your heart rate and blood pressure.

Another procedure that has also been made available is called a vagotomy. This is where the vagus nerve gets cut as a form of therapy. This method has been used for decades mostly as a treatment for peptic ulcers, as by doing this procedure, doctors were able to reduce the peptic acid that the stomach was producing. The vagotomy has slowly been weaned away from being a first option in treatment, however, as it was found to have far too many adverse effects on the system in the long term.

Nowadays you are far more likely to find people having treatment on their vagus nerve in the form of an electrical simulator that is placed in the chest, much like a pacemaker. These electronic devices are able to stimulate the vagus nerve if and when needed in order to treat various chronic medical problems. These vagus nerve stimulation devices have been used to successfully treat severe epileptics as well as severe depression when patients were unable to use drug therapy as a means of medical treatment.

The companies that are making these vagus nerve stimulation devices are now looking into the possibilities of their usage for stimulating weight loss, easing fibromyalgia pain, and combating those nasty migraines that you just can't get rid of. This will be a very promising project for the future once there is solid evidence of it working and being a safe method for each of these medical ailments, but in the meantime we can look out for this magic that the future will bring.

The vagus nerve also serves a very interesting purpose when it comes to the flight or fight mode that our bodies go into when something is wrong. Stimulation of the vagus nerve can result in relaxation after a situation that has left us feeling overly stressed or trapped in that fight or flight mode.

It will also indicate to us when we are in potential danger and need to keep our guard up and our wits about us, keeping us safe in the long run like an animal's instincts would. During emotional stress, if the vagus nerve is overstimulated, it can overcompensate for the sympathetic nervous system and ultimately cause a vasovagal syncope as your heart rate can suddenly drop. It is said that vasovagal syncope is more likely to affect women and children than it does men, and can often lead to loss of bladder control in the moments leading up to an extreme fear or stressful situation.

Because the vagus nerve has efferent fibers that pass through the pharynx as well as the back of your throat, it therefore becomes responsible for your gag reflex, as well as having these nerve endings going straight down the esophagus. The stimulation of these receptors can potentially cause vomiting and in the long run, if overstimulated, may also result in a vasovagal response as discussed earlier.

The functions of the vagus nerve in the gut also play an interesting role. These nerves allow a feeling of being satiated once you have eaten a meal. If the vagus nerve is damaged or blocked, the receptors can then cause you to take in far more food than what is needed and it will then end up causing hyperphagia.

The Autonomic Nervous System

The autonomic nervous system is a part of the nervous system that controls bodily functions that are we are not consciously aware of or controlling ourselves. In order for us to understand the autonomic nervous system, we need to know that the nervous system is made up of two opposing systems that are constantly sending information back and forth the brain and back to the organs.

The sympathetic side of the autonomic nervous system is mostly in control of your energy levels, alertness during the course of the day, your blood pressure, breathing, and heart rate.

This part of the system prepares us to act when it is needed and greatly affects hormones that give you your fight or flight reactions, namely adrenaline and cortisol levels. The parasympathetic side of the nervous system which contains most of the vagus nerve's functions and which the vagus nerve is greatly a part of, is there to decrease alertness, help with calming effects on the body, lower your heart rate and blood pressure, as well as aid your body with relaxation in stressful moments and help with digestion. Because the vagus nerve is a large part of the parasympathetic system, it also plays a role in helping with urination and defecation as well as sparking sexual arousal!

You can picture these two systems working together much like the accelerator and brake in a car.

The sympathetic nervous system would be your accelerator and it gets us up and going with all the energy in the world, and then when it comes time to calm down and relax, the parasympathetic nervous system will be your decelerator and will therefore reduce the speed at which we are going, and will then use certain neurotransmitters such as acetylcholine in order to lower your blood pressure and heart rate and cause the organs of the body to slow down their processes, too.

Chapter 1 The Vagus Nerve

Imagine that your body is a country and you want to explore it starting from a major city and heading south. You stop to see all the sights and important cultural destinations. Sometimes you stick with one road and then turn back when the road ends. Then you choose another road to follow. When you travel like this, you often take branches off the main road, maybe explore some of the little side lanes, and maybe make a lot of U-turns! Eventually, you come to the end of the road, and the end of your wandering, but never the end of your adventure. This road map is similar to your nervous system.

Your nervous system has routes that start from your major "cities": your brain (cranial nerves) and your spinal cord (spinal nerves). Cranial nerves start from your brain and go in all sorts of directions, just like a road map from a big city. There are cranial nerves that only go short distances, and nerves that go great distances. For example, your optic nerve goes a very short distance, from your brain to your eyes. It gathers the information from your retina and sends it back to the vision center of your brain, which then interprets the data. That is how you understand what you see. All of your cranial nerves stop somewhere interesting in your body and relay the information that is there back to the brain. Without these cranial nerves, we wouldn't be able to understand what we see, hear, feel, smell, or taste.

What Is the Vagus Nerve?

The nerve that wanders the most, from the brain to the lower body, is the vagus nerve. In fact, its very name means 'wandering' since it travels from the brain all the way down to the colon. It is the longest nerve that is a part of your autonomic nervous system. The wandering vagus nerve is your connection between your brain and how your body feels. When people tell you to "listen to your body" or "follow your gut," they're basically telling you to listen to and follow your vagus nerve. But that doesn't flow off the tongue quite as easily. Your vagus nerve is incredibly insightful! In an infinite loop, the vagus nerve interprets your environment and sends signals to your organs to act in a specific way. Likewise, your body's reaction can then tell the vagus nerve what is happening in your environment, which causes it to react again. And so on and so on in a never-ending loop. Your vagus nerve is vitally important to understand your own mental and physical well-being, and understanding how and why your body reacts a certain way in a specific environment.

What Does It Do?

Like all good things, the vagus nerve is multipurpose. While the optic nerve only handles one thing (interpreting sight), the vagus nerve juggles so many different aspects of your body. The most important thing it does is connect your brain's understanding of environment and experiences and translate that into responses from your major organs like your heart, lungs, and gastric system. It impacts all aspects of how you respond to different stimuli. Let's look at some examples.

On any given Friday or Saturday night, you're probably going to go out with friends. For this example, imagine that these people are your close friends, not just acquaintances or the new guy from work. When you first walk into the restaurant or your friends' home, your body immediately starts to change. Your heart rate slows, and your breathing deepens. You feel warm, comfortable, and can easily understand your friends' facial expressions. You're fully engaged with what is happening and respond to their actions with similar ones. Your body language is more open and you feel a sense of freedom. Your facial expressions probably match the facial expressions of your friends, and you generally feel safe. At this moment, if you take the time to listen to your body, you'll be aware of all of these reactions. Your body's response to this environment and these people is all due to your vagus nerve. It regulated your heart rate, created the feeling of safety, helped you become socially engaged by understanding and reflecting the emotions around you, and helped your body relax. The experience of being with loving, safe people resulted in your vagus nerve creating loving, safe reactions in your body.

When you say goodbye to your friends and start your long walk home in the dark, your body will start going through different reactions. The warmth that you felt before will begin to dissipate, and as the loneliness seeps in, your heart rate will increase. On a dark, lonely walk home, you may become hyper-focused to what's around you. If you hear someone walking behind you, your breathing may increase, your heart rate may increase, and you may start feeling a little twitchy. Depending on your past experiences, the area you live in, or even depending on the experiences of others like you, your body may slowly start to go into flight or fight response if you hear someone walking behind you. You may feel anxious, and your palms may start to sweat.

Every horror movie or story you've ever heard before will start to replay in your head as you continue walking home. Every shadow may seem to jump out at you, and every footstep behind you may seem infinitely louder. All of this is your vagus nerve reacting to your past experiences and connecting with your current environment. It's warning you of danger, whether there is an actual danger or not. Your sweaty palms, rapid heartbeat, and accelerated breathing are not because of your vagus nerve's actions but are rather because of its inaction. Your vagus nerve helps you feel calm and safe, so in situations where you might feel like you're in danger, your vagus nerve responds with, "Why yes, you are in danger, so I won't stop your body's necessary reaction." Essentially, your vagus nerve decides to sit back with some popcorn and see what comes out of the situation, rather than trying to calm you down. While it's an automatic response, there are things you can do to restore calm and change your vagal response.

This scenario is one of mild stress, but it can quickly become severe stress if you've had previous, terrifying experiences in the dark. Your vagus response can be completely disengaged if your brain and body feel like they're about to experience trauma. This is the fight, flight, or freeze response of your body.

From the examples above, we can see that your vagus nerve affects your physiology or your body's responses. We can also see that it can affect your mental responses too. Let's take a closer look at how the vagus nerve works with your body and mind.

Effects on physiology

The wandering vagus nerve touches many of your major organs, and because of this, it controls a lot of sensory and motor actions for those organs. The major systems that the vagus nerve affects are your cardiovascular system, your digestive system, and your respiratory system.

Your cardiovascular system is like a mail sorting system. Except, of course, it's a life or death mail sorting system. It deals with how your blood gets around your body, and how your blood delivers packages of necessary items like oxygen, carbon dioxide, and nutrients to each cell. The vagus nerve deals with your heart and blood pressure, two things that are critical to life and your cardiovascular system. In the examples mentioned earlier, you may have noticed some physical effects for each of the situations. There were signs like a slowed heartbeat while feeling safe. During signs of distress, there were opposite actions like increased heart rate. These differences are because of how your vagus nerve affects your heart. The vagus nerve can slow down your heart rate and lower your blood pressure. So in times of safety, your vagus nerve is actively keeping you calm and your heart rate low. In times of perceived danger, your vagus nerve steps back and lets your body increase your heart rate. In your cardiovascular system, your vagus nerve is responsible for keeping things low and steady.

Your vagus nerve is also closely connected with your digestive system. The moment you eat food, you are using your digestive system. From your esophagus, down through your stomach and liver, and ending at your colon, your digestive system is responsible for processing the food you eat, and turning them into nutrients for your body or waste to be discarded. Your vagus nerve touches many parts of your digestive system. It connects with your stomach and regulates the release of digestive juices that break down your food. It also regulates the contraction of muscles to move food along and connects with your liver and pancreas to release hormones to help with the nutrient use. Additionally, your vagus nerve helps signal to your brain when you are still hungry and when you are full.

If you're familiar with watching or even reading crime dramas, then you'll probably remember the multiple detectives saying, "I know there's no evidence, but I'm following my gut," or something similar. Everyone in the show roles their eyes until the detective is proven right, and their gut is vindicated. You've probably also experienced something. You might call it intuition, or following your own gut when making decisions. But did you know this is an actual thing? Following your gut is absolutely correct! Your gut literally tells your brain things that influence your emotions based on the environment (Klarer et al., 2014). And the way it gets its message across is with the vagus nerve. Your gut is a strange, sensory organ and is very intimately connected with the outside world and the inside body. Because of this connection, your gut, or rather your gut microbiota, can actually detect and sense changes, and it sends these warnings to your brain via the vagus nerve. Your brain's reaction might be one of fear, anxiety, relaxation, or a changed mood. Either way, your gut and your vagus nerve work together to help you make emotional decisions.

The final system that your vagus nerve affects is your respiratory system. This is your body's way of getting oxygen to your cells and includes your obvious organs, the lungs. The vagus nerve helps your lungs regulate each breath. This means it helps determine the timing of your inhales and exhales and how much you are inhaling and exhaling. In the examples before, there were two different types of breathing pattern experiences. The first was slow, deep breathing when you are in a safe place with safe people. The second was quick, shallow breathing when you are in a questionably unsafe environment. This is your vagus nerve responding to the two different environments. In the safe one, it is telling your body to relax. But in the unsafe environment, your vagus nerve disengages and lets your adrenaline and cortisol take care of everything.

Your vagus nerve is critical in many of your body's systems, but there are other ways that it affects your physiology:

- It activates the pharynx and larynx to help with swallowing and speaking.

- It's connected to your gag reflex, which is why if you don't have one, it could be a sign of a malfunctioning vagus nerve.

- It's responsible for reactions like sneezing, coughing, and vomiting.

- It can suppress inflammation in various areas of your body by controlling the release of anti-inflammatory chemicals.

If your vagus nerve isn't fully functioning, then you might have difficulty in all of these areas. You may have cardiac arrhythmias or an inconsistent heart rate. Your blood pressure may also be inconsistent, being too low or too high. You may faint a lot or more frequently because of the changes in your heart rate and blood pressure. You may have some digestive issues with bloating, pain, vomiting, or nausea. And finally, you may see changes in your voice quality or even your ability to speak at all.

Effects on mental health

The effects that your vagus nerve has on your mental health are closely related to how it works within the autonomic nervous system. Your autonomic nervous system controls your automatic, unconscious bodily actions. Within the autonomic nervous system are three parts: the enteric, sympathetic, and parasympathetic systems. For this discussion, we'll focus on the sympathetic and parasympathetic systems. These two parts of the autonomic nervous system work together in perfect balance. They provide your body with key responses to different environments. The sympathetic nervous system is your 'flight-fight-freeze' response system and your parasympathetic is your 'rest and digest' system. Both of these systems can affect your mental health and well-being.

The 'flight-fight-freeze' response is your sympathetic nervous system's response to terrifying or stressful experiences. Fight and flight often occur together. In this situation, you may feel a certain amount of helplessness and stress. There can be a lot of fear and anxiety involved. Your physiology changes, and your body starts preparing to escape the situation. Our lives are already fairly stressful and often, the sympathetic nervous system being overactive can lead to increased anxiety or depression. In the freeze response, everything is increased and the anxiety becomes extreme. This usually comes around because of trauma and can result in PTSD with recurrent freeze states in non-dangerous situations. This is where your vagus nerve comes in.

Your vagus nerve is the main nerve for the parasympathetic nervous system and is all about calming you down. The parasympathetic nervous system is called the 'rest and digest' system for a reason. When your vagus nerve is functioning correctly, your body will be calm and in a state of rest. When your sympathetic nervous system engages, your parasympathetic system and vagus nerve should also activate to help calm you down again once you're safe. However, if this doesn't happen, then you remain in a state of anxiety, which leads to difficulty with mental health and well-being. Later in this book, we'll explore some struggles we all go through and how we can activate our vagus nerve and parasympathetic system to bring our body back to a state of calm.

One thing that can be very surprising is that even minor fears can be interpreted as an actual danger by your vagus nerve, resulting in disengagement. That's why your heart races during a presentation or job interview. It's why you start to sweat or feel anxiety in situations that are not life-threatening. This is your sympathetic nervous system activating and your vagus nerve refusing to engage. In these situations, you can always try to 'restart' your vagus nerve to help you calm down.

Here is a chart that spells out our physical and mental reactions to the sympathetic nervous system in comparison to when our vagus nerve is engaged in the parasympathetic nervous system.

	Rest and Digest (Parasympathetic)	Active (Beginning of Sympathetic)	Fight/Flight (Sympathetic)	Freeze (Sympathetic)
Situation	Safe, calm, relaxed	Alert to environment	Danger	Threat to life

Cardiovascular State	Heart rate and blood pressure are normal	Increasing heart rate and blood pressure	Fast, strong heart rate, and high blood pressure	Very fast heart rate and blood pressure is very high
Digestive State	Normal or increased	Decreased digestion	Digestion stops entirely	Digestion stops and the bowels and bladder release
Respiratory State	Breathing is normal and steady	Increasing breathing with breaths becoming shallower	Quick and shallow breaths	Very quick breaths with little air being inhaled
Social State	Safe and willing to	Probably willing to	Focused more on	There is no

	connect with others	connect with others	the environment and less on possible social connections	awareness of others or self; unlikely for social engagement
Emotional State	Calm, relaxed, feeling love or sexual arousal	Anxiety, anger, excitement, shame	Fear or rage	Terror or even disassociation from the experience

Adapted from Rothschild, 2016.

From this chart, we can see how the parasympathetic system is very different from the sympathetic one. When the vagus nerve is activated, it doesn't matter what state you are currently in, it will start to calm you down. However, there can be one negative. If you are in a 'freeze' state, and there doesn't seem to be an end to the threat, your body can activate the parasympathetic system in order to prepare for death. When this happens, you start to lose awareness of everything and completely disassociate from the experience. Your heart rate and breathing rate drop to dangerously low levels as your vagus nerve prepares your body to escape the situation in the only way it can. This only happens in periods of extreme trauma or reliving/rethinking about extreme trauma.

Your sympathetic nervous system and your outside experiences can all influence your mental health for the negative. If in a place where you finally feel safe and calm, your vagus nerve can be activated to bring you back to a state of calmness and relaxation.

Since the vagus nerve is so important, it's easy to become really worried about its functionality. If you're a little anxious to begin with, your brain might be screaming at you, "What if our vagus nerve isn't functional?!?" Cue horror movie soundtrack. However, you don't have to panic. While you won't be able to determine functionality at home, your doctor can. Even if you have a perfectly functional or a malfunctioning vagus nerve, there are a lot of things you can do to help regain or improve functionality. If your vagus nerve is not functioning well, your doctor may give you a device for external stimulation of the nerve. Or they may recommend a more invasive, pace-maker like device for stimulating the nerve. There are also some non-invasive, non-medical treatments that can help, which we'll discuss in this book.

To conclude this chapter, what the vagus nerve does is critically important to functionality. Whether or not it's functioning well can affect how you respond to regular, everyday stimuli. In general, the vagus nerve and its response are fairly stable throughout your adult life, but you can always improve functionality. You can take actions that can hack your vagus nerve by using your body to send different messages to your brain and improve your vagus nerve functionality.

Chapter 2 Natural Ways to Stimulate Your Vagus Nerve

Regular stimulation of your vagus nerve will keep it working well and will improve vagal tone. Like muscles, the nerve requires regular exercise to keep it toned and to function at its best. While diet and being grateful can help your vagal tone, there are quite a few other ways to stimulate the nerve.

You don't need to use all of the methods explained below. In fact, you can stick to just one or two, if you like. There are a number of options here, but what is important is that you take steps to stimulate the vagus nerve. That means selecting activities that you enjoy or are comfortable with. Gradual changes tend to stick better than an abrupt, complete lifestyle change, so choose just one or two things to add into your routine first. Then you can gradually add on from there.

Improving your lifestyle is a big step and it can be difficult to really make it happen. Don't let this be another resolution that you start and then drop. It's far too important for that, especially if you suffer from health problems related to the vagus nerve malfunctioning or being damaged. You can improve your symptoms, but you need to actually do the work in order for that to happen.

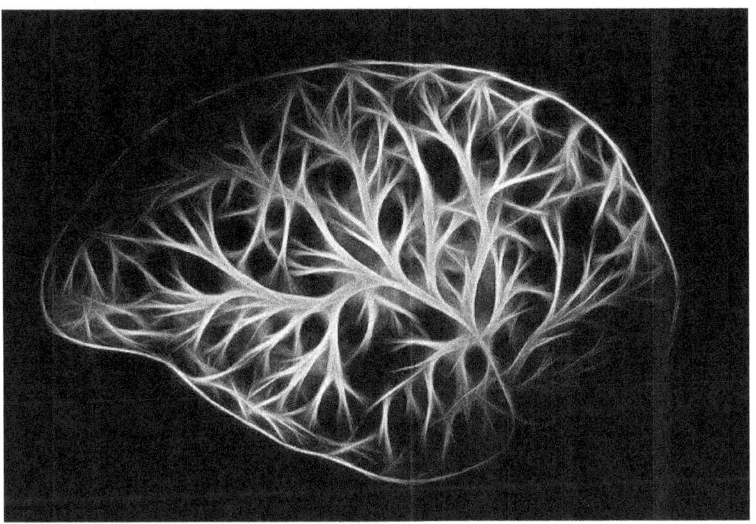

Exercise

Everyone knows that exercise is good for them, but you may not have considered that it actually aids your nervous system. We tend to think of exercise as something we do for our muscles and physical health, but it is just as useful to our mental health.

Once I learned about the effect of exercise on the vagus nerve, I started forcing myself to walk every day, even when it hurt. Sometimes I only got around the block. Sometimes I managed a few blocks. The idea was to keep moving and to keep exercising.

Any kind of exercise can be beneficial, so pick something you enjoy. If you like the exercise you're doing, you will be more likely to keep it up. A few activities you might like to try include:

Walking: Just a stroll around the park or the block can help boost your activity level.

Swimming: This is a good low-impact exercise for those with limited mobility and it builds muscle tone, too.

Cycling: Jump on a bike and start pedaling to boost lung capacity, lose weight, and tone your nervous system.

Hiking: This is a good option for getting into your social connections, too, since hiking is best done with a friend or two.

Running/jogging: You don't have to run a race (though that's fun, too), but getting out and moving fast will give you a vagal tone boost.

Weight lifting: If going places isn't something you enjoy, try weight lifting to tone both muscles and the vagus nerve.

Yoga: Build tone with stretches and add in some social elements, too, if you take a class.

Aerobics: Another great way to get moving is with an aerobics class, or you can do a video class at home.

Dancing: Who doesn't love dancing? Hit the clubs or just stay home and dance your way around the house. It all counts.

Kayaking: Get out on the water and get some exercise for a relaxing vagal tone increase.

Martial arts: You can learn to defend yourself and boost your vagal tone at the same time.

Gymnastics: You will learn to stretch and move, so it's a two for one kind of deal.

Sports: If you enjoy playing basketball, soccer, or something else, you'll find that playing a sport on a team gives you a real energy boost.

There's no limit to the types of movement you can try. If something doesn't work for you, move on to something else.

If you find that exercise is tough for you to keep up with, even when it's something you enjoy, there are a few ways to ensure you keep it up. There's nothing wrong with a little added motivation to keep you moving.

Find an accountability partner. Working out with someone else, even if it's just a walking partner, is particularly helpful. If you make a date to meet with someone to exercise, you'll be more likely to keep the date, rather than bailing at the last minute. Alternatively, you can just have someone that you report to each day, even if they're long-distance. Having to check-in will give you more reason to do what you said you would.

Sign up for classes. If you spend money on classes, you'll likely keep up with them. After all, you wouldn't want to throw away the money. Just make sure it's something you actually want to do. It makes little sense to take a karate class if you hate martial arts, for example. There are so many different physical classes available that there's no shortage of things to learn.

Join a team. Really need some motivation? Consider joining a sports team. Whether you want to play baseball locally or jump into dragon boating, a team will keep you going when you don't feel like moving, simply because there are other people depending on you. For those who are competitive, a team sport can be very enjoyable and may get you moving even more than usual.

Hire a trainer. A personal trainer is an extra expense, but if you can afford it, you'll have someone to push you to your limit. I found that a personal trainer really helped me get past the exercise hump. When I couldn't push myself, it helped to have someone else there to push me.

Get a dog. Not only does a dog make a great companion and give unconditional love, but it will also need to be walked. You can't get away with skipping the walks or you'll have a mess in your house. The extra motivation to go out might be just what you need to get moving.

It can also help to reward yourself once you reach a certain goal, such as running a distance in a certain amount of time or lifting a certain amount of weight. You choose your reward, but it should be something that will motivate you.

Vocal Exercises

Since the vagus nerve has pathways extending to your vocal cords and into the throat, vocal exercises can be beneficial. The vibrations activate the vagus nerve and help build your vagal tone.

What exactly are vocal exercises? Anything that engages the throat can count. Actual talking is one option, but you can also hum, chant, sing, or gargle to activate this area of the vagus nerve. Anything that moves the vocal cords or the muscles at the rear of the throat can stimulate the nerve and improve its function. Doing this on a daily basis can help improve vagal tone drastically.

Try singing in the shower each morning, or as you prepare for the day. It's great for your nervous system, but it also helps put you in a great mood. If you have to drive to work, you can crank the music and enjoy a singalong as you drive.

Another option is to learn to chant. You can find recordings of inspiring chants that are meant to help you feel empowered and strong. Just like with singing, you can use these on your daily commute, or whenever you have a little time alone. The same goes for humming or making other noises. Enjoy it, get into it, and reap the benefits.

Interact Socially

Positive social interactions have been shown to cause the activation of the vagus nerve, which means you need that interaction with other people. Even introverts can benefit from talking to someone else, sharing a meal, or engaging in activity that is shared with another person, or multiple people. However, it is important that these interactions remain positive, since negative interactions and relationships can actually lower vagal tone.

When interacting with someone else, there are a few ways to increase the vagal tone benefits for both of you. First, establish a meaningful, connected relationship with the other person. This will help both of you. Making eye contact and physical connection can also be beneficial. Hugs are a terrific way to stimulate the vagus nerve, thanks to both physical pressure and positive associations.

You've probably noticed that when you get a hug from someone, it just feels really good. Some people are better huggers than others, but the connection strengthens with hugs and physical contact, making it more likely that you'll continue the relationship and view it in a positive light. All of this is good for your vagal tone and should be pursued whenever possible.

Look After a Small Child

Mothers get a rush of hormones immediately after birth, including oxytocin, which helps them bond with their child. This is the same hormone that is released with positive social interactions. Parents can benefit from being in close contact with their babies and children, but even if you don't have a child, you can experience the benefits.

Researchers have found that caregiving can actually stimulate the vagus nerve and improve its tone. Looking after small children is an excellent way to get this started, plus you're likely to get lots of hugs and sloppy little kisses. All that physical contact is bound to help with your vagal tone. Babysitting is a good way to get a little dose of caregiving.

Not one to enjoy children? While babies and toddlers are excellent for your vagus nerve, you can get that caregiving bonus from looking after animals or older people, as well. Try volunteering at a nursing home, as a respite worker, or in another position where you can help look after someone or something. This will help you release more oxytocin, improve your vagal tone, and you'll be doing something wonderful for the world, as well.

Cold Exposure

You may have heard that cold showers or dips are good
for you, but did you know the cold actually activates
your vagus nerve? It also affects the cholinergic
neurons along the vagus nerve. Cold exposure will
stimulate the nerve and help tone it, making it more
efficient.

You can reduce stress or anxiety by reducing the
sympathetic nervous response to stressors. Cold
exposure can boost parasympathetic activity, which
helps bring down the fight and flight response. It can
also help reduce stomach issues. If you feel sick, being
exposed to cold can often reverse the feeling of nausea
that you feel.

Methods of cold exposure vary. There's the infamous
jumping into an icy lake, but something a little more
attainable would be to take a cold shower or even
splashing cold water on your face. You might start off
slow by just turning your shower to cold for the last
minute or so and gradually work your way up to a
completely cold shower. However, you decide to do it,
you'll notice the improvements in your health in a few
weeks.

Some people enjoy going outside in the winter without bundling up and this can be an excellent way to add some cold exposure to your life. Even a few minutes can affect your vagus nerve and improve things for you.

Studies have shown that cold on the neck is the most effective, so try putting a cold washcloth on the back of your neck for best results.

Laughter

They say laughter is the best medicine, and it's true. In fact, it's entirely possible that the person who coined the phrase was actually referring to stimulating the vagus nerve. That's exactly what laughter does. A hearty belly laugh hits the vagus nerve at multiple points, including the throat, chest and even the abdomen. It's a massage for your organs and your nervous system and will boost your vagal tone.

The best part about laughter is that it is something easy to do and quite enjoyable. A lot of adults lose the ability to laugh at every little thing, but if you watch a child, they break out into giggles constantly throughout the day. It's a feel-good thing to do and a great habit to form.

Start by enjoying something humorous. Watch a comedy show online, read a funny book, or take turns telling jokes to a friend or child. You'll soon find yourself cracking up and enjoying a boost in both mood and vagal tone.

Make a point of laughing every day so you can give yourself that internal massage and stimulate the vagus nerve. We should all have the opportunity to laugh at least a few times in a day. If you're not, then it's time for some changes in your life.

Massage

Certain types of massage can stimulate the vagus nerve. Reflexology has been shown to stimulate the vagus nerve and improve both vagal tone and reduce anxiety. Foot massages can lower the fight or flight response and engage the vagus nerve, but other types of massages are also beneficial. This is a very physical method of stimulating the vagus nerve and it can be terrifically effective if you use it right. Besides, who doesn't enjoy a good massage?

Your massage can be in just one area of your body or you can go for a full body massage. Have a loved one do it for you or get a professional to stimulate that nerve. Whatever you choose, make sure it's relaxing and enjoyable. If you hate having your feet touched, for example, you're not going to get as much benefit from a foot massage as you would if you enjoyed it.

Face massages that include the neck are excellent for stimulating the vagus nerve, but even a good shoulder massage from a friend can give you the benefits you're looking for. If you need an excuse to have more massages, now you have it. It's all for your vagal tone.

Chiropractor

Your body needs to be in good condition in order to release the vagus nerve and tone it. If you have any blockages throughout your body or if you are out of alignment, it can affect the overall tone of the nerve.

A good chiropractor will be able to treat any blockages that the nerve might have and release it. You'll find that it is much easier to tone your nerve when it is unblocked, so a visit to the chiropractor from time to time is a good idea.

Sex

We have a sex drive for a reason and aside from reproductive purposes, sex can be an excellent way to stimulate the vagus nerve. Any activity that engages the pelvis, such as Kegels, can be used to activate your vagus nerve and sex is the ultimate way to engage the pelvis and stimulate the various nerve endings found there.

However, sex isn't just about pleasure and orgasm, though these are very good ways to boost vagal tone. When you engage in intercourse or even just foreplay, with someone, you are engaging in social interaction and a very intimate method of connecting with another human being. This can gives you a double whammy when it comes to vagal tone and can cause you to feel happier and calmer overall.

Of course, this doesn't mean you should engage in sex with anyone. Even self-pleasuring techniques can give you half of the equation and help boost your vagal tone. However, if you have a special someone to enjoy intimate time with, you'll definitely notice the benefits over time.

Enemas

When you think of stimulating the vagus nerve, enemas probably aren't the first thing that comes to mind, but they can be very effective. After all, the vagus nerve is particularly affected by the gut and so if you activate it, you activate the vagus nerve.

When you insert liquid into the rectum, your body must hold it in. This exerts control over your body and activates the pelvis, which also activates the vagus nerve. Resisting the urge to defecate is actually very helpful in toning the vagus nerve, so enemas can be useful for this purpose, but the type of enema is also important.

Coffee can be used to give yourself an enema that will stimulate the vagus nerve. Any liquid will help with this, but coffee is best, because it contains compounds that actually stimulate nerve endings. In addition, it gets the bile ducts flowing, which helps with digestion.

Enemas in general, as well as those with coffee, help flush toxins out of the bowels, too. This reduces inflammation and helps improve vagal tone. You can make your own enema from cool coffee, or you can buy pre-made enemas in bottles that are easily used. If you make your own, stick to one teaspoon of coffee grounds per enema, as it can be too strong to use full coffee.

Acupressure and Acupuncture

Acupuncture and acupressure are very similar, apart from the fact that one uses pressure and the other uses very thin needles to stimulate specific pressure points. Both methods allow you to physically stimulate the vagus nerve and enhance the parasympathetic reaction. It's considered a good alternative to the implant that we looked at previously.

By inserting needles or adding pressure to specific points in the body, it's possible to stimulate the vagus nerve and rapidly improve its tone. This is something you can do at any practitioner's office and they should be well aware of which points to use in order to open up the nerve's function.

Each of these methods can be done easily and will not cause you further harm. If you are serious about activating your vagus nerve, I highly suggest you select three or four of these activities and schedule them into your daily routine. It shouldn't add too much time to your day and the results can be incredible.

Chapter 3 Measuring Nervous Function with Heart Rate Variability (HRV)

We saw earlier what the HRV is all about. This time, we are going to take a closer look at the concept and how it can be used to measure the functioning of the vagus nerve.

An important thing to note is that the HRV is a non-invasive method of measuring the Autonomic Nervous System (ANS).

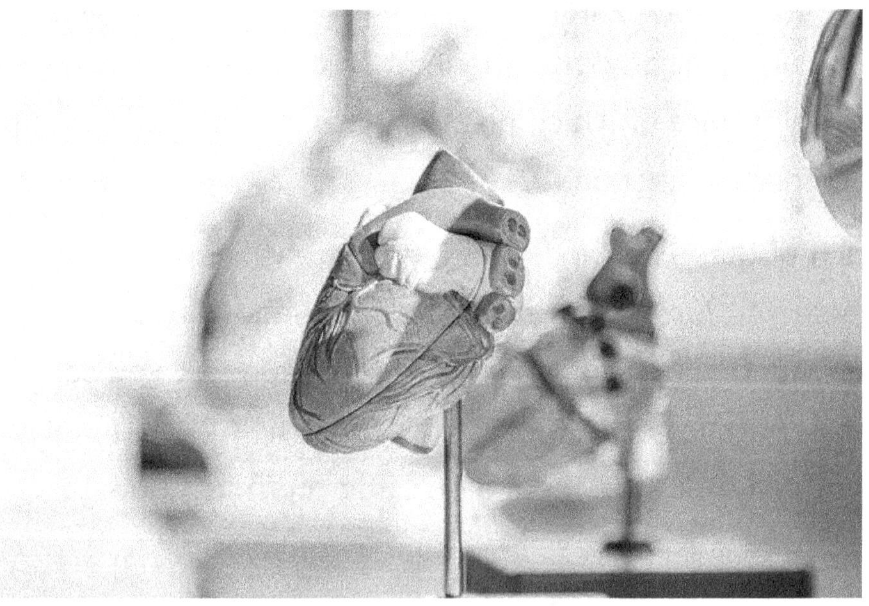

Typically, the heart rate of a person is used to understand a lot of factors. A high heart rate typically means that the person has a high blood pressure or might be suffering from anxiety. But when you use

HRV, you get a more accurate understanding of how the Autonomic Nervous System is functioning. Here are some of the things that you can understand using HRV:

- How well you recover from stress

- The body's resilience and ways to improve it

- Optimizing physical training and recovery of the heart from anxiety and other situations

- Help with sleep and nutrition

- Improve mental health–mood, depression, anxiety

- Improve mental performance and cognition

- Identify risk of diseases

- Measure the inflammation rate in our bodies

- Bring balance to the nervous system

- Discover any changes to the health and well-being of the person

Think about it. We can get a whole lot more data about the nervous system when we make use of the HRV. It is like opening a big encyclopedia and finding out the information that we require.

But just how is this related to the vagus nerve?

Think of the above scenarios for a moment. In fact, let us take the first point, how well you recover from stress. We have seen the many contributions of the vagus nerve towards stress. The fact that the vagus nerve can help the body release more happy chemicals helps us combat bad mood and poor mental health. But imagine having more accurate data about the way in which we recover from stress and if the rate of recovery is fast or too slow. With that data, we can see how effectively our vagus nerve is functioning. Slow recovery means that there is something we are doing wrong. It could be poor diet, poor condition of the vagus nerve, or simply our daily habits. Even if the vagus nerve was helping us, but our stress levels are high, then it is an indicator that we might have to incorporate some of the routines that we had talked about before. Every bit of information gives us a clearer picture of how effective something is and if there is another problem that we need to look at.

Now look at the other points and you will see the same scenario played out with them. For example, improving the body's resilience relates to the body's immunity.

Our vagus nerve helps with our immunity. After all, it is through proper digestion (assisted by the vagus nerve), that we have enough good nutrients in our body, which eventually go towards keeping our body energized and our immune system active.

As you go through the rest of the points, you begin to get a clear picture of the importance of HRV for measuring not just the body's condition and health and mental status, but also how well our vagus nerve is functioning.

In fact, the HRV is directly used to gauge the Parasympathetic Nervous System's fight-or-flight response. By understanding more about the response, we are able to discern:

- Increased fitness level

- Better health

- Better resilience

- Youthfulness

- Willpower

- Calm and positive emotions

With a lower HRV, we know that the fight-or-flight response has been affected. Through that, we can understand the below:

- Reduced fitness level

- Poor health

- Increased disease risk and inflammation

- Faster aging process (where we feel the effects of age quickly). For example, you might have seen people who are barely in their mid-thirties and either suffer from diabetes or effects like lethargy. On the other hand, you might have seen people who are above 60, but have great energy and youthfulness about them. All of this depends on how well you can take care of your vagus nerve

- Negative emotions

- Increased anxiety and depression

HRV is indeed a good measurement of our overall health and our vagus nerve condition.

Chapter 4 Substances That May Interfere with the Vagus Nerve

It is good to know about the many foods that help you improve the vagus nerve. It helps you manage your diet and change your eating habits.

But that is just one part of the equation. There is the part where we are thinking about adding more of something and then there is the part where we have to reduce some of the good stuff. Think about it. It does not matter how many salads and greens we eat if we only end up heading over to KFC and ordering a nice 10-piece chicken bucket.

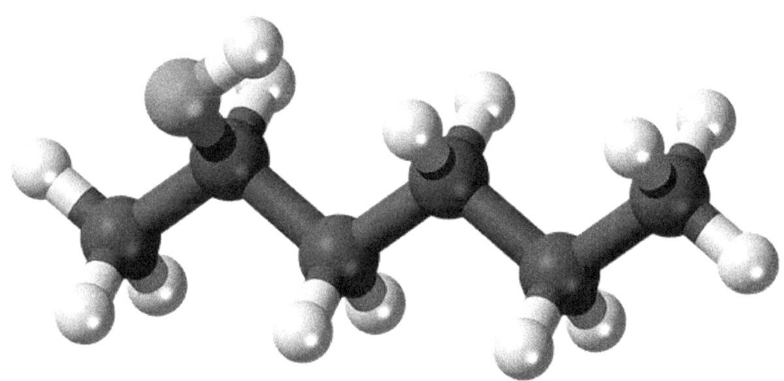

The same principle applies to the vagus nerve as well. We need to swatch what we eat, both by including healthy food and removing harmful components.

Apart from the food we eat, we also need to watch out for other substances that enter our bodies. While you might think that these substances do not have any effect on the vagus nerve, you might be surprised by the results.

Let us look at some of these substances.

Breathing is essential for life. We take in oxygen that fills up our lungs and gets carried into our blood. We exhale carbon dioxide, by-products of a successful breathing process.

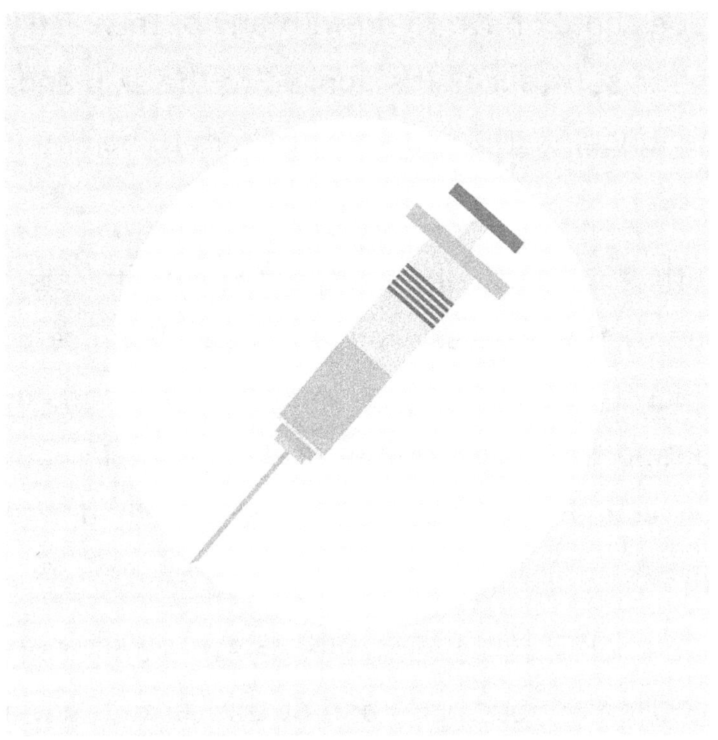

But what exactly tells our body to breathe? Is it our mind? Our brain?

Well, our brain is definitely involved, but there is much more to breathing than that. You see, what tells our lungs to not stop breathing and suffocate us is a certain neurotransmitter called acetylcholine. Guess what part of the body is responsible for the creation of these neurotransmitters? That's right. It is the wonderful vagus nerve that we have come to fondly adore (by now I hope that is the case).

What does botox have to do with any of this? Isn't that a cosmetic substance? It's applied to the skin and not into the lungs, so there does not seem to be any connection.

The truth is not in the process, but the chemicals released by the process. You see, when you use botox, you inject the stuff into your muscles. This ends up interrupting the production of acetylcholine in your body. Which is why botox can be potentially dangerous to you.

Too much botox can eventually lead to a deficit of acetylcholine in your body and at the same time, a blockage of the vagus nerve. The only conclusion to all of this is the end of our lives.

While that might sound grim, it is a reminder of how to maintain control over what you do. It helps you to understand that some things should not be taken in excess.

Certain Antibiotics

Now I am not telling you to completely stop taking antibiotics.

When you have a certain strain of bacteria affecting your body and causing all sorts of damage, then you need antibiotics to deal with the situation. In short, listen to your doctor.

But at the same time, the name says it all. Antibiotics attack the bacteria in our body. The way they do this means they don't focus on getting rid of just a particular bacteria, but related bacteria as well. This is why they could cause harm to some of the useful bacteria that live in our body.

That still does not mean that you have to skip out on the antibiotics. So what else can someone do? Is there an alternative?

This is where probiotics come into play. The main purpose of probiotics is to add useful bacteria into the body. This becomes useful when you are consuming antibiotics. For example, let's say that a particular antibiotic has removed a certain bacteria from the body. Using a probiotic replenishes that particular bacteria.

Doctors are careful about this and usually prescribe probiotics to their patients if the need arises. However, remember that if probiotics are not needed, then you don't have to ask for one. Your doctor is usually aware of the risks of prescribing certain antibiotics and if he or she feels that you might need to take something else along with your medications, then that is usually given to you. If you feel doubtful, always ask your doctor for more clarification. They would be happy to explain to you.

Heavy Metals

Heavy metals, like arsenic, lead, mercury, and others, are all around us. They're in the ground we walk on, in the water we drink, and in the products we use every day. But high levels of most heavy metals can make you sick.

When you get a high dose of a certain heavy metal, then you might suffer the symptoms below:

- It might disrupt your brain functions and you might end up feeling lost or confused.

- Numbness in certain parts of the body

- Nausea and vomiting

- In certain instances, you might pass out completely.

How does mercury harm the vagus nerve? Well, let's just say that you could consider botox and mercury as partners in crime because they both operate the same way; they affect the production of acetylcholine in the body. This in turn prevents the body from sending proper signals to the lungs to breathe.

Is there a way to prevent mercury poisoning? Of course there is.

Keep in mind that trace amounts of it might be found in numerous food that we eat and that low levels are usually ignored or managed without difficulty by the body. But some of the foods that you can avoid in order to prevent a higher level of mercury in your body are:

- Fish that has high levels of mercury

- Any additional supplements or dietary pills with high mercury

Excessive Sugar

Excess sugar is bad for a lot of reasons. Apart from the fact that it is one of the biggest causes of diabetes, it is also harmful because it causes chronic inflammation. Such inflammation creates disruptions on the body's cellular feedback loops and other signaling pathways. What this means is that different parts of the body are not able to communicate with each other well. Of course, communication is the primary function of the nervous system.

It is also for this reason that when high amounts of sugar cause blurry vision, difficulty thinking, and fatigue, the body thinks that you are getting a panic attack and falsely activates the fight-or-flight process. But the reality is that you are not having a panic attack. Your body does not realize this because it is taking time for one part of the body to tell the other that it's just a false alarm.

In order to prevent such disruptions in communication, make sure you reduce the intake of sugar. If you are someone who cannot keep away from that delicious Hershey's bar of chocolate, then either choose to have it in moderation or, in the case of diabetes or any indicators of diabetes, you have no other choice but to skip it entirely.

Chapter 5 Vagus Nerve Stimulation

The thought of going to the hospital or seeking some form of treatment usually feels us with dread. They are synonymous with pain and suffering, and while no one likes going to the doctor, we all get infections or ailments from time to time that requires medical care and treatment. However, there are ways that we can tap into the natural self-healing power of the body and reduce the number of times that we need to seek medical intervention,

Diseases are a natural part of life because our bodies are susceptible to the wear and tear that comes with age as well as infections and physical damage inflicted by pathogens and other stimuli. This means that the quest for good health is a never-ending journey because we cannot escape the inevitable effect of nature and our surroundings on our health.

Whether you find your comfort at the bottom of the pill bottle, or in alternative therapies, our goal ultimately remains the same; to improve our quality of life by staying healthy and avoiding diseases. The quest for longevity has led to the development of research in various aspects of medicine, from disease prevention, diagnosis, treatment, and cure, the winding road to better health has led to important findings that we can use to better our health.

While human advances in medicine cannot be downplayed, it is important to remember that medicine has side effects on the body. When taken for prolonged periods of time, conventional medicine can have adverse effects on our bodies in the form of side effects. While conventional medicine is beneficial for the treatment of various ailments and conditions, we should do the necessary to reduce the incidences where we need to take it and avoid over-reliance on pills and potions.

In an ideal situation, being able to stimulate the vagus nerve effectively will enable the body to become more adept at keeping illnesses at bay, meaning that you will need less medical intervention to stay healthy. The body's self-healing mechanism functions best when the internal environment is in a rested state.

This means that when the fight and flight responses are activated, the body's self-healing mechanism cannot work. Therefore, when you unleash the parasympathetic power of the vagus nerve through stimulation, you effectively shut down the fight or flight responses and activate the body's self-healing mechanisms.

The 10th cranial nerve, which is the Vagus nerve, is the longest nerve in the body extending from the brain through the neck and thorax all the way to the gut. This nerve, with its sensory and motor response functions, has significant roles in the regulation of organs such as the heart, lungs, and gut. The parasympathetic roles of the vagus nerve, which inhibit the effects of the sympathetic nervous system, meaning that the vagus nerve is an important factor for proper organ function and optimum physical and mental health.

The roles of the vagus nerve in maintaining homeostasis and balance in the internal environment of the body have led to the discovery that the vagus nerve can be used not only in boosting our overall immunity but also in facilitating the body's self-healing mechanism.

Now that we can appreciate how important the vagus nerve is when it comes to good health, the next question would be, how do you measure the activity of the vagus nerve? That is where the vagal tone comes in.

Vagal Tone

Vagal tone is the term used to refer to the activity of the vagus nerve.

heart rate regulation

vasodilation and constriction of vessels,

glandular activity in the heart,

glandular activity lungs

gastrointestinal sensitivity and motility and

regulation of inflammation.

When it comes to health, the vagal tone is measured in terms of the consistent nature of the parasympathetic action that the vagus nerve exerts. While the vagal input is constant, the degree of the stimulation it exerts is influenced by various factors including the parasympathetic responses of the autonomic nervous system. This means that the vagal tone will vary depending on the internal environment in the body. For instance, when the body is in a state of fight or flight, then the vagal tone or activity will be diminished.

Vagal tone can be used as an indicator of various organ functions in the body, including cardiac function, and may also be used in assessing emotional regulation or any other factors that can be influenced by parasympathetic responses such as digestive functions.

The measurement of vagal tone is done using either invasive or noninvasive procedures. Measurement of the vagal tone using invasive procedures is characterized by the use of manual or electrical methods to stimulate the vagus nerve. When it comes to non-invasive techniques, the vagal tone is typically determined by the assessment of the heart rate and heart rate variability. Heart rate variability (HRV) is the difference in the time lapse that occurs between heartbeats.

When the vagal tone is high, then the heart rate is typically slower, and on the other hand, an increased heart rate is an indication that vagus nerve activity is diminished. The vagal tone in the body is a useful tool in the determination of emotional, psychological, and even possible physical disorders that may manifest as a result of poor vagal activity or function.

☐   Vagus Nerve Stimulation

The vagus nerve has both afferent and efferent functions in connecting the brains to organs such as the heart, lungs, and gut. This means that it facilitates communication from the brain to the organs (afferent) and communication to the brain from the organs (efferent).

The vagus nerve functions in controlling motor responses in the voice box, diaphragm, heart, and stomach. In addition, it has sensory functions in the ears and tongue. The widespread nature of the influence on the vagus nerve on different organs, therefore, makes it a useful treatment therapy in patients with diseases caused by chronic inflammation, including Alzheimer's, Epilepsy, and Rheumatoid arthritis.

When Vagus nerve stimulation therapy is to be used on a patient, a device that is similar to a pacemaker is implanted in the chest of the patient. A wire from this device is then run from the device to the vagus nerve in the neck by making incisions on the left side of the neck, which allows for the wire to be placed beneath the skin. This device then functions by sending electrical impulses to the vagus nerve which, in turn, transmits these signals to the brain.

These pulses that are transmitted to the brain are used in the treatment of patients with conditions such as drug-resistant depression. The impulses help in battling depression by affecting the circuits in the limbic system of the brain, which is the area that is responsible for our moods and emotions.

In epilepsy, vagus nerve stimulation therapy works in a similar manner. The signals transmitted from the implanted device travel to the vagus nerve, where they are then sent on to the brain. These mild electrical pulses sent to the brain help in controlling the abnormal brain activity that causes epileptic seizures. While vagus nerve stimulation therapy does not cure epilepsy, it plays a big role in reducing the frequency, duration, and severity of epileptic seizures. This therapy has become an important tool in the management of epilepsy.

Perhaps one of the most incapacitating illness, that is caused by chronic inflammation in the joints is rheumatoid arthritis. Not only does it result in severe joint pain, but rheumatoid arthritis also restricts movement as well, and may lead to joint deformities in the long run. This disease is challenging for patients because it severely affects the quality of life by limiting the independence of the sufferer. It has no cure meaning that the patient needs to learn to limit and slow down the degeneration in the joints.

Vagus nerve stimulation therapy has proven to be useful in the management of the inflammation that causes joint degradation, and as such, helping in slowing down the course of rheumatoid arthritis and minimizing symptoms such as joint pain and swelling. When the vagus nerve is activated, it releases acetylcholine and inhibits the production of the tumor necrosis factor from the pancreas.

Both of these mechanisms initiated by the vagus nerve are effective in the reduction of inflammation, and therefore, offer relief in terms of the level of inflammation in terms of swelling, pain, and deformation of the joints. In rheumatoid arthritis, vagus nerve stimulation therapy can be invasive, as in the case of surgically implanting a device to function as a pacemaker or non-invasive where the vagus nerve is stimulated externally.

Vagus nerve stimulation therapy has been used in the treatment of patients with gastroparesis. Gastroparesis is the condition where food movement through the gut is inhibited, resulting in food staying in the stomach too long and blockages being formed. This disease can lead to bacterial infections, abdominal pain, bloating, loss of appetite, and weight loss. Vagus nerve therapy functions by innervating the muscles in the digestive tract that facilitate the movement of food in the digestive system through peristalsis.

These are all classic examples of situations where vagus nerve therapy is used in conjunction with conventional medical intervention to realize quicker treatment or aid in alleviating symptoms that do not necessarily respond to medical pills. However, vagus nerve activation is not only useful for people who are already sick. This nerve can help you in maintaining and improving your physical health and mental state, and as such, we can all benefit from the self-healing powers of this powerful nerve that makes up part of the body's self-healing mechanism.

Activating the Vagus Nerve

The good news is that you do not need to have a device surgically implanted in your body to access the healing powers of your vagus nerve. Your vagal tone is the indicator of the activity of your vagus nerve, meaning that if your vagal tone is high, then the level of activity of your vagus nerve is high, and if the vagal tone is low, then the vagus nerve activity is equally low.

While you might wonder why this vagus nerve is so significant, it is important to realize that in our bodies, like in everything else, too much of anything is detrimental. If you are constantly anxious or revved up in fight or flight mode with a flood of adrenaline coursing through your veins, sooner or later, this will take a toll on your heart, mental state, and overall health.

Conditions such as chronic inflammation, depression, or chronic anxiety arise from an inability to switch off the sympathetic responses and restore calmness and balance in the body. Your vagus nerve is one of your most important tools in achieving a relaxed or rested state that allows our organs, tissues, and body to operate without stress, and hence, achieve optimum functional levels physically, mentally, and emotionally.

Being on the lookout for symptoms associated with poor vagus nerve functions such as chronic stress and anxiety, irritable bowel syndrome, inflammation, insomnia, chronic fatigue, or hormonal imbalance, can give you an indication of whether or not your vagus nerve is functioning properly.

These symptoms, even when they do not directly arise from poor vagus nerve function, can all be alleviated or prevented to a large extent by stimulating the vagus nerve. The vagus nerve equips us to respond to emotional, psychological, and physical symptoms that arise from a lack of balance or homeostasis in the body.

The two arms of your autonomic nervous system, the sympathetic system, and the parasympathetic system are meant to balance out in terms of function to facilitate homeostasis in the body and ensure that the nervous system is working properly. While the sympathetic system is crucial in enabling us to cope with stresses both external and internal through fight or flight responses, the parasympathetic system is crucial in restoring our body back to a relaxed state after the resolution of stresses.

Phases of alertness that are typical in flight or fight responses that are triggered by the sympathetic nervous system are ideally meant to alternate routinely with periods of rest and relaxation that are typically initiated by the parasympathetic nervous system. This balancing act works by ensuring that we do not remain in either a sympathetic/agitated state or a parasympathetic state/relaxed state for too long.

This ideal situation of equilibrium between the parasympathetic and sympathetic systems is, however difficult to achieve because we live in a world where we are constantly faced with emotional, physical, and mental stresses. This means that our sympathetic nervous system is usually constantly activated to help us deal with the constant stresses we encounter on a regular basis.

When the sympathetic system is consistently overstimulated, it means that the parasympathetic system, including the Vagus nerve, becomes inhibited, and thus we need to find ways and tools that we can use to activate or stimulate the Vagus nerve to effectively switch off the sympathetic system.

As we have already established, the vagus nerve is an important part of the parasympathetic system that helps in restoring body function to normal and mitigating the effects of overstimulation of the sympathetic responses which can lead to conditions such as chronic inflammation, depression, poor stress management, and a host of other complications.

Chapter 6 The Vagus Nerve and Bipolar Disorder

When you have been diagnosed with bipolar disorder you may find that you want to reject the diagnosis, or you may find that you are overwhelmed with the idea of suffering from this illness. However, knowing that you have bipolar disorder is just one step in getting the help that you need.

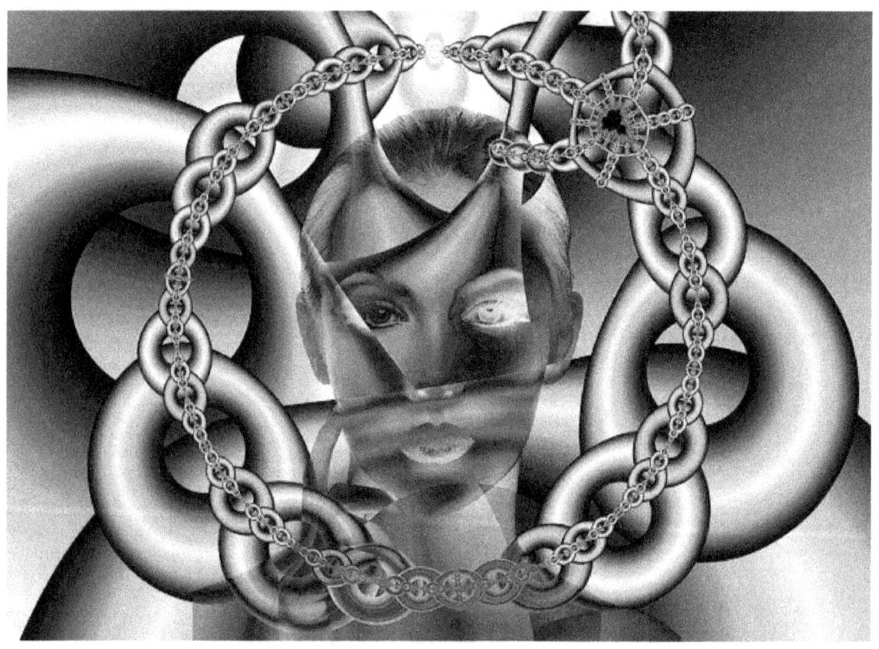

What Is Bipolar Disorder?

Those that suffer from bipolar disorder are going to suffer from extreme mood shifts. This mental disorder can cause a person to feel extremely high highs and extremely low lows. When the person has a very

82

elevated mood it is known as mania however, this person will also experience times of extreme depression as well. Bipolar disorder has also been called manic depression as well as bipolar disease.

When a person suffers from bipolar disorder, they may struggle with day to day tasks that need to be done. They may have a hard time at work or at school. They may struggle to maintain relationships. While there is no cure for bipolar disorder, there is a treatment available.

Almost 3 percent of all adults in the US have been diagnosed with bipolar disorder. That means that about 5 million people in the US alone suffer from this mental illness. The average age of diagnosis is 25.

In order for a person to be diagnosed with bipolar disorder, they have to suffer from depression that lasts for no less than 2 weeks. They also must suffer from manic episodes that last for days or weeks at a time. Some people with bipolar disorder will suffer from mood swings very often while others only suffer rarely. There are those who will spend most of their time in a depressive state and then there are those that will spend much of their time in a manic state.

Some people learn how to manage their symptoms, especially those that rarely experience an episode of mood swings while others struggle every day.

There are three symptoms that a person with bipolar disorder can suffer from. The first is mania. This is when a person feels emotionally high. The manic episode can cause the person to be full of energy. You may notice that they talk faster than normal and have lots of exciting and new ideas. They may start a lot of new projects and seem impulsive. The person feels euphoric when they are in a state of mania. However, this can lead to irresponsible behavior such as having unprotected sex with multiple partners, using drugs, or going on spending sprees.

Those that suffer from bipolar but do not have severe mania suffer from what is known as hypomania. When a person who has bipolar suffers from hypomania, they will still be able to go to work and do well in school. They will also be able to maintain their personal relationships however; they are going to be able to notice a shift in their moods.

A person with bipolar disorder is also going to suffer from depression episodes where they may feel hopeless, extreme sadness, a lack of energy, needing more sleep than normal or the inability to sleep, thoughts of suicide, and they may I lose interest in the activities that they used to enjoy.

While bipolar disorder is not rare, it is very hard to diagnose because the symptoms vary so much.

Men and women both suffer from bipolar disorder equally however, the symptoms that the two experience are a bit different. Most women who are diagnosed with bipolar disorder are diagnosed in their 20s or in their 30s. They tend to have much milder mania and spend more of their time in depressive episodes. Women tend to experience rapid cycling which is when they have more than four episodes in one year. They also tend to suffer from other conditions such as anxiety disorder, obesity, thyroid problems or migraines at the same time they are suffering from bipolar disorder episodes.

It is believed that women relapse more often because of the hormonal change that they experience during menstruation as well as pregnancy, and menopause.

Men, on the other hand, are often diagnosed with bipolar disorder much earlier in life, they tend to have much more severe episodes especially when it comes to mania. It is more likely that a man who is suffering from bipolar disorder will have issues with substance abuse than a woman and it has been found that men tend to act out more when they are having a manic episode. Men are also less likely to seek medical attention when they suffer from bipolar disorder and it is more likely for them to die of suicide than it is a woman.

Types of Bipolar Disorder

There are three different types of bipolar disorder known as bipolar 1, bipolar 2, as well as cyclothymia.

A person with bipolar 1 disorder will have suffered from at least one episode of mania. They may also experience hypomania as well as depressive episodes both before and after they have a manic episode. Bipolar 1 affects both men and women at about the same rate.

Those who suffer from bipolar 2 are going to experience at least one depressive episode that lasts no less than two weeks. They will also have no less than one hypomanic episode that lasts at least 4 days. Bipolar 2 disorder is much more common in women than it is in men.

Those that suffer from cyclothymia are going to have both depressive and hypomania episodes. The episodes are often shorter and not as severe as those that are experienced in bipolar 1 and bipolar 2 disorders. A person who has cyclothymia may go a month or even two while having stable moods.

If you have bipolar disorder, it is important for you to remember that you are not alone. There is help for you and there are plenty of things that you can do in order to improve your life. One that may help is stimulating your vagus nerve.

Bipolar Disorder and Stimulating the Vagus Nerve

Many people who suffer from bipolar disorder do not get the relief that they are looking for from medication. This is very common if they are being treated for both mania and depressive episodes. It is well known that the medications that are provided for bipolar disorder simply make some people feel as if they are not themselves. Therefore, we see so many people stopping their medication and therefore relapsing into a manic state which often gets them into a lot of trouble.

However, because bipolar disorder involves depression, vagus nerve stimulation can be used in the exact same way that it is used for depression. Of course, you can get the vagus nerve stimulation implant that we talked about earlier in this book however, since it costs tens of thousands of dollars that may not be an option for everyone.

The good news is that there are plenty of other ways for you to stimulate your vagus nerve which we are going to talk about later on in this book. You do not have to go into surgery and pay thousands of dollars in order to get a stimulator placed into your body. However, if your doctor feels as if this would be a good option for you, it is possible that your insurance may cover the cost. Depending on how badly your bipolar disorder is affecting your life, this may also be something that you want to consider.

However, it is important to note that if you dedicate yourself to stimulating your vagus nerve on your own, you really don't need one of these devices. By stimulating your vagus nerve, you are going to see the same results as someone who suffers from depression. Your moods are going to stabilize, and you are going to be able to focus on the tasks that you need to get done each day. You will see improvement in your life as well as in your moods.

While stimulating your vagus nerve can help to improve your bipolar disorder symptoms it is very important that you do not stop taking or lower your dose of medications without your doctor's approval. If you are starting to feel better or are noticing that your medications are affecting, you differently talk to your doctor and explain how you are feeling. They may decide that it is time to lower your dosage or even begin to tapper you off from the medication altogether.

Chapter 7 The Lungs and How the Vagus Nerve Affects Them

Years ago, the idea of stimulating the vagus nerve to improve health started with the idea that vagus nerve stimulation would help reduce seizures. Today we are starting to understand just how many areas of our health are affected by the vagus nerve.

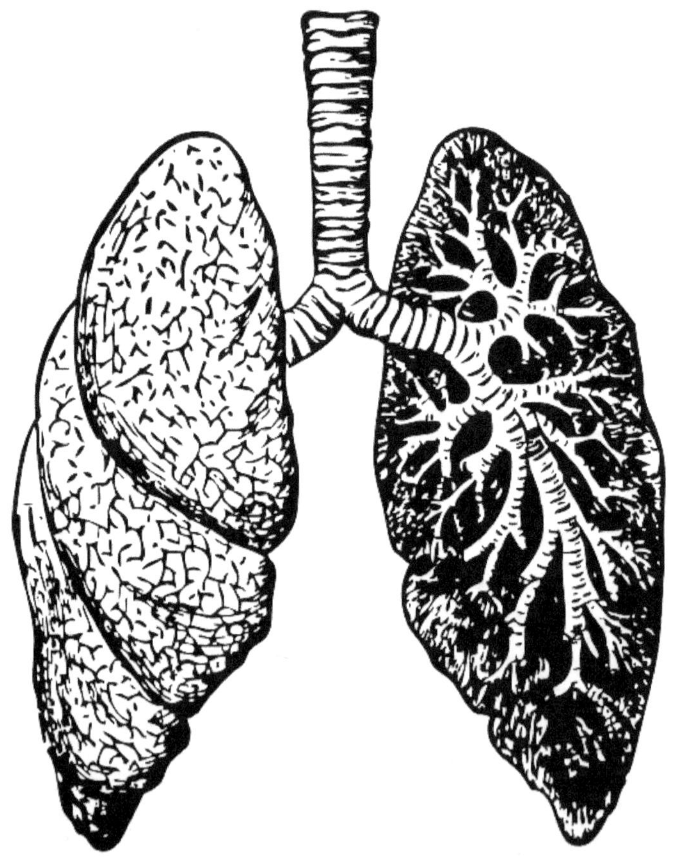

Researchers have found that not only can seizures be treated by vagus nerve stimulation, but depression, bipolar disorder, obesity, strokes, Crohn's disease, and even asthma may be treated as well. Of course, this list could go on and on because every day doctors are finding out that by stimulating the vagus nerve we can improve our health in yet another way.

You see, when you think about the vagus nerve, think about a huge electrical wire. If you cut that wire in half, you are going to find that it is made up of many other little wires. Those little wires in the vagus nerve are going to lead to the different areas of the body that are affected by the vagus nerve. When that nerve is stimulated, each area that wire runs to is affected.

According to the ALA (American Lung Association), there are 1.8 million visits to the ER each year as well as 3,816 deaths reported due to asthma alone. Asthma is a health condition that is long-term and is not curable however, the goal for all asthma patients is to control the symptoms of asthma so that they can live a long and healthy life.

Often times doctors will refer to asthma as chronic respiratory disease. This disease will cause a person's airways to become inflamed and then narrow which makes it hard for them to breathe. It is common for a person who has asthma to cough, wheeze, experience shortness of breath or even chest tightness. When a person has severe asthma, it can make it very hard for them to be active and it can frequently make it difficult for them to talk.

Asthma is a very dangerous and serious disease that does not get the respect that it should. How often do we hear someone say that they had an asthma attack and brush it off as nothing? How many times have we had someone tell us that they have been diagnosed with asthma and we do not think of it as a life-threatening disease? The truth is that asthma can and has taken many people's lives.

Asthma affects every area of a person's life. It can affect their ability to do certain types of work, be in certain environments, and even cause them to be unable to do simple tasks at home. Asthma can be so bad that simply having a conversation or laughing can cause a person to suffer.

Asthmas severity is ranked by its symptoms. Asthma is mild intermittent if the person suffers from symptoms less than two times per week and less than two times a month. This person is going to have very few asthma attacks.

It is considered mild persistent if they have symptoms from three up to six times a week during the day and three to four times a month at night. It is at this point that asthma may start affecting their activity levels.

Moderate persistent asthma is when a person suffers more than six times a week during the day and more than four times per month at night. The person who has asthma will notice that their activity level is affected.

Severe persistent asthma is when a person suffers from symptoms both day and night, most of the time. The symptoms are happening so often that activities have to be limited.

There are different types of asthma. Adult-onset asthma happens when you begin suffering from asthma as an adult. While asthma can happen at any time in a person's life, most people begin to see symptoms before the age of 40. However, if someone in your family has asthma, eczema, or allergies, you are more likely to develop asthma.

Status asthmaticus is an asthma attack that is prolonged and will not respond to normal treatment such as bronchodilators. These attacks need emergency medical treatment immediately.

Children who have asthma may display different symptoms such as coughing a lot when they are laying or laughing or at night. It is possible that coughing will be the only symptom that they display. They may also lack energy when they are playing or have to stop and catch their breath. You may notice that they are breathing shallowly or rapidly. The child may complain that their chest is hurting, or you may be able to hear them wheezing. This sounds as if they are whistling when they are breathing.

It is also possible that you will notice the chest rising and falling more than normal when they are breathing. The muscles in the neck and chest may tighten and the child may complain of being tired.

Exercise-induced asthma happens when a person is moving. You do not have to have any other type of asthma to suffer from exercise-induced asthma.

Allergic asthma is triggered by allergens such as pollen, dust, or pet dander. It causes severe asthma attacks as well as coughing spells.

Nonallergic asthma happens due to extreme weather. This can show up when it is really hot in the summer or when it is cold in the winter. You may also suffer from attacks when you are under a lot of stress or when you have a virus.

When you have an asthma attack several things happen. You may suffer from airway obstruction. This happens because the muscles that surround your airways tighten and the air is not able to move in and out of your lungs. This is what causes shortness of breath and wheezing. Inflammation of the bronchial tubes will cause it to be difficult for you to move air in and out of your lungs as well. However, inflammation can cause further damage to the lungs and it is very important that while you are treating asthma you are treating the inflammation as well.

When a person suffers from airway irritability from for example an allergen, the airway will overreact which will cause it to tighten therefore causing an asthma attack.

While there are lots of treatments out there, from inhalers to pills, to shots, and even surgery, there is no cure for asthma. The damage that is caused by asthma can lead to future lung problems, therefore, it is important to always take your medications.

However, there is more that we can do. By stimulating the vagus nerve we are able to help open up the airways and improve breathing. This does not mean that you should stop taking your medications. You do not want to stop taking your asthma medications without a doctor's approval. However, you can reduce your symptoms and reduce your need for a rescue inhaler by focusing on stimulating the vagus nerve.

The best way for a person with asthma to stimulate the vagus nerve is through deep breathing exercises which we will cover a little bit later. Not only are these going to stimulate the vagus nerve, but they are also going to help improve lung functioning and increase your blood oxygen levels.

Asthma can be scary but there are steps that you can take to reduce your symptoms. You can start right now with vagus nerve activation and stimulation.

Chapter 8 Measuring the Vagus Nerve Tone

Vagal tone is assessed by measuring your heart rate along with your breathing rate. The pulse rate accelerates a little when you breathe in and reduces somewhat when you breathe out. The greater the disparity among your pulse rate of inhaling and your heart rate of exhaling, the lower your vagal tone.

Vagal Tone

Initiating the parasympathetic sensory system is relevant after using the vagal tone. The estimation of your vagus tone is done after having a consistent follow up of your breathing rate. What happens is that, when you breathe in, your pulse rate speeds up and it stops for a short while when you are in the process of breathing out. When there is a great difference between your breathing in and the breath out pulse, there it causes your vagal tone to be high. A high vagal tone means that your body can loosen up in a fast way after pressure.

What Is a High Vagal Tone Related To?

There is an improvement of the capacity of many-body frameworks by a high vagal tone, which causes a great glucose structure, low levels of stroke, also, cardiovascular illness, lower pulse, improved processing by using a good creation of stomach fundamental and stomach related chemicals, and diminished migraine. There is a connection to having a great stable state of mind, which encompasses a low feeling of nervousness, as well as strength when the vagus tone is high. The vagus nerve has an amazing role of going through the gut microbiome and begins to cause an adjustment in order to curb irritation dependent on whether it distinguishes pathogenic versus non-pathogenic living beings. Due to this, the microbiome of the gut has an impact on the disposition, the anxiety feeling, and large aggravation.

What Is a Low Vagal Tone Related To?

Lower vagal tone is associated with cardiac problems and strokes, grief, hypertension, chronic fatigue disease, intellectually disabled, and much higher rates of offensive conditions. Provoking disorders to include all nervous system disorders (rheumatoid joint pain, provocative bowel disease, endometriosis, immune response thyroid disorders, lupus and more).

How Would We Increase Vagal Tone?

Throughout the article mentioned, a device that energized the vagus nerve extended the vagal tone. Luckily, you do this all by yourself, but it requires ordinary training. Rather, you're hereditarily susceptible to changing levels of vagal tone, but this still doesn't mean you can't change it. Here are a variety of different ways to treat the vagus nerve:

Easy, enunciated, diaphragm calming. Inhaling from the abdomen, as compared to shallow breathing from the peak of the neck, activates the vagus nerve.

Murmuring. Since the vagus nerve is associated with the vocal ropes, murmuring precisely invigorates it. You can murmur a tune, or far and away superior recurrent the sound 'OM'.

Talking. Correspondingly talking is useful for vagal tone, because of the association with the vocal lines.

Washing your face with virus water. The instrument her isn't known, yet chilly water all over invigorates the vagus nerve.

Reflection, particularly attentive to the meditation of good will, which promotes feelings of selflessness for oneself and others. Researchers who did a review in

2010 found that increasing positive emotions caused increased social proximity and enhanced vagal tone.

Improve the microbiota of the abdomen. The presence of strong microscopic organisms in the intestine gives the vagus nerve a pleasant feedback ring, widening its sound.

The implications on your overall well-being of these clear and basic behaviors, and especially on frustration, are comprehensive. If by any chance of feeling the negative effects of a troublesome disease, agitated stomach-related, hypertension or suffering, it is deeply recommended to take a quick look at the vagal tone. We have understood for a considerable period of time that meditation and reflection are valuable for our well-being but familiarizing ourselves with the process through which they operate is so mesmerizing. I am sure that this brief article has encouraged you to begin a practice of meditation, as it is for me, and to look for specific with the ability of the body to deal with reactions.

Polyvagal Theory

The polyvagal hypothesis clarifies three distinct pieces of our sensory system and their reactions to distressing circumstances. When we comprehend those three sections, we can perceive any reason why and how we respond to high measures of pressure. If polyvagal hypothesis sounds as energizing as watching paint dry, stay, trust me. It's an entrancing clarification of how our body handles passionate pressure, and how we can utilize various treatments to change the impact of the injury.

What Is the Importance of the Polyvagal Theory?

For specialists, and pop-brain science aficionado the same, understanding polyvagal hypothesis can help with: Getting injury and PTSD, Understanding the move of assault and withdrawal seeing someone, Seeing how outrageous pressure prompts separation, or closing down, Seeing how to peruse non-verbal communication, We like to think about our feelings as ethereal, complex, and hard to sort and recognize. Truly feelings are reactions to a boost (inward or outer). Frequently they occur out of our mindfulness, particularly in the event that we are distant, or incongruent, with our internal enthusiastic life. Our basic want to remain alive is more critical to our body than even our capacity to consider remaining alive. That is the place the polyvagal hypothesis comes in to play. The sensory system is continually running out of sight, controlling our body capacities so we can consider different things—like what sort of dessert we'd like to request, or how to get that an in-prescription school. The whole sensory system works pair with the mind and can assume control over our passionate experience, regardless of whether we don't need it to.

Let Us Look at an Example of the Case Before We Dive into the Actual Discussion

Creatures are an extraordinary case of how we handle pressure, since they respond basely, without mindfulness. They do what we would, on the off chance that we weren't so all around restrained. In the event that you have ever viewed a National Geographic Africa extraordinary, you've seen a lioness pursue a gazelle. A gathering of gazelles is brushing, and all of a sudden one gazes upward, hyper mindful of what's going on around him. The entire gathering notification and focuses. After a minute, the lioness begins her pursuit.

The gazelle she's singled out keeps running as quickly as possible (thoughtful sensory system) until he is gotten. When he is gotten, he in a flash goes limp (parasympathetic sensory system).

The lioness hauls the gazelle back to her whelps, where they start to play with it before they go in for the slaughter. On the off chance that the lioness gets occupied, and the gazelle sees a snapshot of chance, he's up and runs off once more, appearing as though he abruptly returned to life (once more into thoughtful sensory system reaction). At the point when the gazelle was gotten, with teeth around his neck, his shutdown reaction kicked in—he solidified. When he saw the chance to run, his battle or flight kicked in, and he ran. The polyvagal theory is based on the three themes, namely: connection shut down and flight. Polyvagal hypothesis covers those three states—association, battle or flight, or shutdown.

Here is How They Perform.

Connection

During non-upsetting circumstances, on the off chance that we are genuinely sound, our bodies remain in a social commitment state, or a glad, ordinary, non-blow a gasket state. This is a connection. By association, I imply that we are equipped for an "associated" connection with another person. We are strolling near, unafraid, making the most of our day, eating with loved ones and our body and feelings feel ordinary. It's additionally called ventral vagal reaction since that is the piece of the mind that is initiated during association mode. It resembles a green light for a typical life. What does this look and feel? Our insusceptible framework is solid. We feel ordinary satisfaction, receptiveness, harmony, and interest in existence. We are resting soundly and eating regularly. Our face is expressive. We genuinely identify with others. We all the more effectively comprehend and tune in to other people. Our body feels quiet and grounded.

Flight

The thoughtful sensory system is our quick response to push that influences almost every organ in the body. The thoughtful sensory system causes that "battle or flight" state we have all known about. It gives us those prompts with the goal that it can keep us alive.

How Does This Occur? What Does This Look and Feel?

We sense to risk and stop to examine the surroundings for genuine threats. We discharge cortisol, epinephrine, and norepinephrine to enable us to achieve what we have to escape or battle our foe. Our pulse spikes, we sweat, and we feel more activated. We feel on edge, apprehensive, or irate. There might be flashes of outward appearances of dread and outrage, with the foundation of all the more a still face. On the off chance that positive feelings are available, they typically look constrained. Our processing backs off as blood hurries to the muscles. Our veins choke to the digestion tracts and widen to the muscles expected to run or battle. We might need to flee, or punch somebody, or respond physically somehow or another, or simply puff-up and look terrifying. Our muscles may feel tense, electric, tight, vibrating, hurting, trembling, and hard. Our hands might be sticky. Our stomach might be horrendously tied. Every one of our faculties focus on it. Our motions may show guarding of our crucial organs such as clenched hands grasped or puffing ourselves up to look greater or more grounded. In battle or flight, at some level, we accept we can, in any case, endure whatever risk we believe is risky.

What's fascinating about this piece of the parasympathetic sensory system? It can keep us solidified as a versatile system to enable us to make due to either battle or flight once more. At the point when David Livingston was assaulted by a lion, he later announced, "it caused a kind of vagueness in which there was no feeling of torment nor sentiment of fear, however very aware of every one of that was occurring." At the point when our thoughtful sensory system has kicked into overdrive, despite everything we can't escape and feel approaching passing the dorsal vagal parasympathetic sensory system takes control. It causes solidifying or shutdown, as a structure self-conservation. (Consider somebody who goes out under outrageous pressure.)

What Does This Look and Feel?

Inwardly, it feels like separation, deadness, unsteady, misery, disgrace, a feeling of inclination caught, out of the body, detached from the world. Our eyes may watch fixed and scattered. The dorsal engine core through the unmyelinated vagus nerve diminishes our pulse, circulatory strain, outward appearances, sexual and insusceptible reaction frameworks. We might be activated to feel sickened, hurl, poo, immediately pee. We may feel low or no torment. Our lungs (bronchi) contract and we inhale slower. We may experience issues getting words out or feel tightening around our throat. Our cerebrum has diminished digestion, and this causes lost body mindfulness, limp appendages, diminished capacity to think plainly, and diminished capacity to set down story recollections. Our body stance may crumple or twist up in a ball. In the mode of the shutdown, at some point, our sensory system accepts we are in a dangerous circumstance, and it attempts to keep us alive through keeping our body still.

Heart Rate Variability

To comprehend HRV, we first need to comprehend our sensory system and pulse. Pulse inconstancy can be followed back to our autonomic sensory system. The autonomic sensory system manages significant frameworks in our body, including heart and breath rate and processing. The autonomic sensory system has a parasympathetic (rest) and a thoughtful (actuation) branch. Pulse changeability is a marker that the two branches are working the parasympathetic specifically.

Inherent pulse is measured in the absence of parasympathetic or reflective guidance. When hampered by autonomous guidelines, strong heart contracts each period at a rate of about 100 pulsates (the amount is as human as this may be). For example, concerning cardiovascular planning, pulse modifiability has been analyzed.

When you start customary cardiovascular preparing, one of the quickest positive adjustments of your body is expanded blood plasma volume, and hence expanded stroke volume. Thus, your heart can keep the blood streaming and keep up satisfactory circulatory strain at a lower pulse. Furthermore, as we recollect, the lower pulse is directed by the parasympathetic branch. Parasympathetic guideline causes longer interbeat interims and raised HRV. In the long haul, normal exercise likewise reinforces the heart muscle, which by and by methods lower HR and higher HRV. All in all, high pulse fluctuation means that particularly cardiovascular, yet additionally by and large wellbeing just as general wellness. As a rule, it reveals to us how recuperated and prepared we are for the afternoon. Additionally, HRV can respond to changes in our body significantly sooner than pulse. This makes it an especially touchy instrument that gives us experiences in our prosperity.

Parasympathetic guideline brings down your pulse from the inherent level, giving more space for inconstancy between progressive pulses. Parasympathetic guideline causes practically prompt changes that influence just a couple of thumps one after another, after which the pulse returns towards the inborn rate. Thoughtful guideline raises your pulse from the inborn level, and there is less space for fluctuation between progressive pulses. Thoughtful guideline influences a few backs to back heart thumps. Pulse inconstancy is one of the pointers of the condition of your wellbeing and wellness, recuperation, and preparation. Be that as it may, your HRV esteems, similar to your general wellbeing and wellness, are a blend of a few things, so focus on yourself and how you feel all in all. HRV is a decent marker; however, it's still only one pointer. Try not to depend a lot on it, or some other measure alone. With that off the beaten path, here are a few different ways you can gain from your HRV esteems.

The main thing to focus on is your very own HRV gauge. That is, your run of the mill HRV when you're feeling as you feel by and large. Your standard is the beginning stage for your HRV investigations. You will get a comprehension of your HRV pattern in the wake of utilizing the Oura ring for some time because Oura indicates you both the daily HRV esteem and the long haul HRV pattern.

In the wake of finding your gauge, you're prepared to catch up on how your way of life and wellbeing influences your HRV. On the off chance that your HRV goes down, something may trouble your body and additionally mind. On the off chance that your HRV goes up, something may do useful for your body and additionally mind.

The Testing of the Vagus Nerve

If you want to check the status of your vagus nerve, you are required to seek the doctor's check-up. They will further examine your gag reflex while using soft cotton to check two sides of the rear part of your throat. The result of this exercise should cause you to gag and the lack of it means that there is a problem with your vagus nerve. So, which are these problems that the vagus nerve may have? By now, you are aware that the vagus nerve CN X is so long and therefore, its impact may be too much because it connects to many areas. There are potential symptoms that will alert you on the damage of the vagus nerve. Looking for a good therapist is determined by the effect that you feel in your body. A good therapist will take you through tests that aim at checking the main problem so that they can recommend medication.

Measuring Vagal Nerve Tone

Vagal tone is the degree of relaxation caused by the vagal nerve. It is mainly a biological process that involves the tenth cranial nerve located in the brainstem's medulla oblongata. For that reason, it is a crucial component of the parasympathetic branch that regulates the homeostasis of body organs. This function is vital as it controls the subconscious body organs such as the eyes, lungs, heart, digestive tract, and the adrenal glands. It is a representation of the index in which the functional state of the vagus nerve is determined. For instance, a vagus nerve with a high vagal tone shows the system can combine body systems and makes them cooperate to benefit the whole body and coordinate in times of harsh response.

The vagal nerve's function to calm the body organ also helps in the relaxation of the gut, pupillary diameter, salivation, and heart rate, creating a calm situation where the body repairs itself. Therefore, the regulation of your emotions and the ability to remain peaceful and quiet is determined by the vagal tone for it is the vagus nerve that induces the calm state of the body. In this case, your nervous system should be capable of handling the signals that will be created to coordinate the experienced consciousness and higher energy, but without a well-functioning and healthy nervous system, the spiritual experience remains muted. The heart rate is controlled by how you inhale and exhale. The heart beats faster whenever you breathe in to quicken the circulation of the inhaled oxygen around the body. On the contrary, the heart rate becomes relatively slower when you breathe out. It is one of the most critical regulations done by the vagus nerve.

The difference between the heart rate when you breathe in and out is the vagal tone. For that reason, the higher the gap, the higher the vagal tone. A high vagal tone is recommended as it regulates the mechanism and amount of sugar in your blood, reducing the possibility of developing diabetes, cardiovascular diseases, and stroke. On the contrary, a relatively low vagal tone has been associated with chronic diseases and inflammation. Inflammation is a way of the immune system to heal an injury and fight off bacteria in body parts and organs. However, it could be damaging to the blood vessel and body organ if it is prolonged or happens for no reason.

The immune system detects an attack on the body and releases protein that causes inflammation. The vagus nerve is responsible for resetting the immune system and inhibiting the production of these proteins. The higher the vagal tone, the higher the effectiveness of stopping the production of this protein. A low vagal tone means that the ability to stop inflammation will be less effective. The effectiveness of your vagal tone must be understood by taking various measurements depending on multiple factors such as your preference. With the following techniques, you will learn ways and reason to perform the task:

Facial observation. These are positions and motions of the muscles found under the skin of your face. The movements shown on the face help the observer understand your emotional state. The psychological aspect of facial expression makes them dependent on the nervous system, so there must be ways in which you could measure the vagal nerve tone for it is a major source of various facial expressions. The vagal tone is the measurable organismic variable that contributes to developmental differences in every individual. The parasympathetic and sympathetic nervous systems regulate the homeostatic function that targets most organs found on the face. The vagal nerve communicates both sensory and motor information to these organs to influence how you make your expressions.

Facial muscles are critical in enhancing the expressions for effective communication between people. The fascia in the face, as well as the connection of the muscles and the skin, play a significant role in enhancing the movements. By moving the skin, the muscles create folds and lines that cause facial movements involving the eyebrows and mouth. The same muscles enable other functions that need stretching, such as chewing.

115

Facial expressions are meant to convey emotions or communicate non-verbal messages to second parties. Some of the emotions that you could make include happiness to reflect the satisfaction, joy, pleasure, and contentment in your mind. It is a popular emotion characterized by an expression making you raise both corners of your mouth upwards.

Disgust expression is associated with infectious, inedible, offending, and unsanitary things. For instance, a person may show this expression if you say or do hurtful things. It is a feeling you expect in revolting experiences and is a common retaliation to anything that elicits the feeling either through appearance, smell, sight, taste, or sound. A disgusted person raises their upper lip and cheeks while wrinkling their nose bridge. The feeling is known to decrease the heart rate. Anger is a feeling associated with a significant range of intense rage and irritation. It is known to heighten the blood pressure as a result of an increased heart rate, which is similar to the emotion that makes the body produce an increased amount of noradrenaline and adrenaline.

Whenever you are exposed to a threatening or frightening situation, you may develop a fight-or-flight response that is associated with anger. Whenever you encounter the imminent danger or threat, anger becomes the dominant emotion to enable a psychological and cognitive response. When angry, a person firmly presses up against their lips and lowering their brows while bulging their eyes. The feeling is similar to fear, which also is associated with dangerous and threatening stimuli. Although anger influences a response to the imminent danger, fear is a survival mechanism that is characterized by avoidance and escape. This emotion involves widely opening the eyes and mouth while raising the brows.

The surprise emotion is a relevant and unexpected event that usually invokes a brief state of being that. It involves dropping the jaw and arching the eyebrows—feelings of disadvantage, helplessness, and loss influence sad emotions. The emotions are associated with quietness, withdrawal, and a feeling of exhaustion. By lowering the corners of the mouth and raising the inner portions of the brows, you express sad emotions associated with misery, melancholy, and sorrow. By observing some of these facial expressions, you could tell the heart rate and the breathing pace of an individual in addition to other aspects that involve the vagal nerve.

Evaluating vagal function through heat rate variability. Heart rate variability (HRV) is the change in the time interval between successive heartbeats. It could be used to evaluate the functionality as well as the efficiency of the vagal nerve tone. Cardiac vagal activity shows how your body adjusts to different environmental changes. It also provides a marker of how your body regulates stress and emotions. HRV represents the oscillation of the heartbeats, thus its relevance in indicating stress and other emotions. The utilization of heart rate variability allows the identification of the essential branch of the nervous that mediates the heart rate.

The connection of the heart to the brain affects the functionality of the vagus nerve through the core integration system integrated into the brainstem nuclei and guided by the medial prefrontal cortex. As a result, the heart rate variability offers testable predictions concerning the vagal function in the body. The fluctuation of the "beat-to-beat" interval creates a suitable basis that provides a reasonable measure of vagal nerve tone. An increased sympathetic regulation reduces the mental effort as well as the influence of the baroreflex. In this case, the heart rate variability is directly proportional to the increase in mental effort. The mental load becomes detrimental whenever the mental effort is moderate. Testing the HRV in different situations helps in determining the highest and lowest rate that can be achieved. This way, the results reflect the efficiency of your vagus nerve as well as your body's compatibility with these functions.

Having relatively low heart rate variability is considered a cardiovascular risk. As you engage in your daily activities, the heart rate changes depend on various factors such as temperature and physical activity. The rate also reflects the changes in demands of the heart that is determined by the moments of anxiety, anger, or excitement. A simple task of breathing in and out changes the heart rate. Medics consider it, as usual, to have the heart rate variability during the day as it shows that the heart is in sync mode with other parts of the body. The variability also indicates the heat's awareness of the requirements in certain parts of the body. A constant heart rate throughout the day could be considered as abnormal and could be a sign that the heart might be somehow stuck at a specific rate.

Although low heart rate variability may not be a disorder, it may serve as an indicator of an underlying condition such as depression. If the condition is left untreated, it may increase the risk of cardiac arrest. Persistent activation of the sympathetic nervous system is a common cause of low HRV. It also makes the heart remain in high gear as the system hyperactively responds to significant depression. Altering the activity of the autonomous nervous system as in the HRV is a significant contributor to the worsening of cardiovascular-related conditions. The variations of the heart rate provide a clear reflection of the cardiovascular control systems to various physiological perturbations. Besides, the fluctuations play a significant role in enhancing respiration.

For that reason, the heart rate variability is a sensitive measure of how the sympathetic and the parasympathetic systems function. It is responsible for measuring the changes that occur in the natural "beat-to-beat" of the heart rate. The evaluation can be done using simple tools and equipment that regulate the coherence and the state of body stress and balance. The coherent heart rhythm reflects positive emotions from individual experiences such as compassion and appreciation. Similarly, the irregular heart rhythm reflects the negative emotions that you experience, including anxiety or anger. These reflections enhance brain functions that result in a significant reduction in cognitive performance, stress reduction, a person-centered approach, and respect-based communication.

Vagal tone through polyvagal theory. The theory by Dr. Stephen Porges explains how different parts of our nervous system respond to various situations. It is useful among psychology enthusiasts and therapists as it helps them understand the mode and course of attack and withdrawal inmost relationships. The theory also explains how shutting down and dissociation are influenced by extreme stress. Therapists utilize the theory to understand trauma and read the body language of victims. The theory eases the difficulty we perceive in trying to understand and categorize emotions and outlines how the nervous system is always responsible for controlling body functions in the background. The system coordinates with the brain to take over our emotional experience and change how we behave in certain situations.

The vagus nerve maintains the connection made that is characterized by a non-stressful and happy state. The status enhances interaction among people through the parasympathetic nucleus ambiguous response. The ventral vagal response ensures that the immune system is healthy and able to detect and counter injuries and infections in the body. At this stage, you feel open, curious, and happy about life as you have nothing to worry about or have no illusion of perceived threats. You enjoy your food and have a good appetite while having no difficulties sleeping. These signs are essential in helping you understand your vagal tone as you noted that even facial expressions tell more about your psychological state. At the connection and restful state, you experience a good relationship with others both physically and emotionally as you can listen to them and understand their perspective even if they may be having different opinions. At this stage, your body feels more grounded and calm and live in the present.

These observations are contrary to what you would expect in case of the fight-or-flight response of the nervous system. The sympathetic nervous system is responsible for activating reactions to stressful or threatening situations. The vagal tone is identified, especially if you are in a frozen state or surrounded by real danger. The body releases norepinephrine, epinephrine, and cortisol to escape from the threat or to fight our enemy. The condition is characterized by mobilization and heartbeat spikes that make you afraid, sweaty, anxious, or angry. The digestive process is slowed down as more blood is supplied to the muscles through the constriction of intestinal blood vessels and dilation of the muscle blood vessels.

The shutdown status is also activated by the dorsal motor nucleus that keeps you frozen to regain the ability to a fight-or-flight response. The condition occurs as a result of the takeover of the vagal parasympathetic nervous system after the sympathetic kicks to overdrive. At this stage, you experience emotional numbness and disconnection from the world. The dorsal motor nucleus decreases the facial expressions, blood pressure, heart rate, immune and sexual response systems. Through the three states, you could understand how your vagal tone responds to the environment and the efficiency through all the body organs. Therapy could also be necessary, especially in people with dissociation episodes and chronic suicidality after subsequent or attachment trauma.

The Importance of Therapists Tests

Some of the psychological disorders do not have a clear cause or treatment. At times, you may experience struggles as you maintain your professional and personal relationships. The best thing would be to seek testing and evaluation to get the best attention and avoid possible incidences in the future. The administration of these tests is done by qualified personnel who have experience in conducting interviews and performing most of the tasks involved in testing and evaluation. In case of diagnosis, the testing clinician refers you to a treating therapist who rechecks the credentials and ensures that you are comfortable being attended by them. Most of these tests are done to find out whether there is an underlying cause of social or behavioral problems.

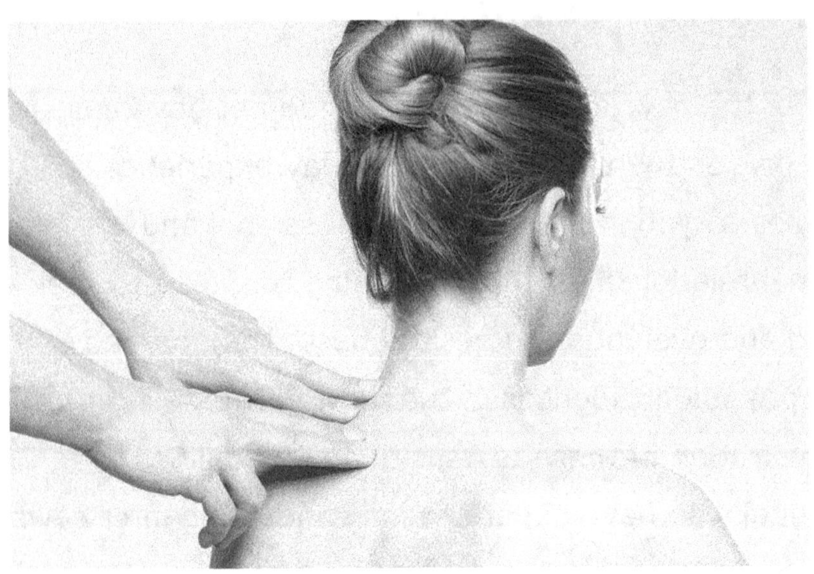

If you have these problems, you are likely to exhibit an attention deficit, learning disorder, or emotional problems such as depression and anxiety. In some of the modern therapist tests, the therapist may decide to rule out some of the conditions that are less associated with the evident behavior. Therapist tests have become a common phenomenon, especially among social workers, employees, and medical doctors. The tests take place in a medical facility and may take several hours in each visit. It may involve questionnaires, checklists, and surveys to evaluate your reflection on various aspects of your life and the world in general.

You do not have to prepare for these tests as you cannot tell what they will be all about. The most important thing is to express frank and transparent opinions and responses to the questions you find, no matter how sensitive they might appear. Testing and evaluation are important for the following reasons:

The results are used to find out whether there are additional health problems that were underreported or not observed. It helps in collectively dealing with all the problems and easing the worries you might have in your life.

It is worth waiting as you need very little time to fill out the questionnaires and respond to direct questions asked by the therapists. It is time-efficient contrary to other types of tests that take longer to be completed.

With these therapist tests, the therapist will assess your ability to handle strong emotions depending on how you view the tests and how you respond to them. Through the testimonial of what you have passed through, the therapist will test your body's capabilities in responding to moods and emotions.

After collecting the relevant information from you, the therapist will make a precise evaluation of how to deal with the underlying causes. Most of the time, the solution to these problems reduces even the physical issues that were caused by a psychological trigger.

Therapist tests are not only meant for survival but are also suitable for the quality of your life. The step-by-step testing and evaluation help in relieving tension in your body as the problem-solving procedures help you develop a positive attitude towards life and the world.

Results acquired from the therapist's tests play a significant role in guiding you in the direction you ought to take to recovery. This way, you will be able to change unhealthy patterns as you untangle many years of confusion and turmoil in your life.

Direct contact with therapists helps you view the condition as solvable, mainly due to the freedom of expression where you are allowed to ask concerning and personal questions. The responses from the professional will help you understand the condition as well as the processes involved in treating it.

It is a primary source of education as you will learn most of the things that your family members or friends know nothing about.

Therapist tests are critical in examining the extent of brain injury or the disorder to decide the best and most effective measures to take to address it.

It is also a critical factor in determining whether you are fit to stand any trial before you.

Through these examinations and evaluations, you can understand what causes social and behavioral patterns. A therapist also measures your body's capabilities to respond to different situation and how the vagal tone affects the response.

Chapter 9 The Polyvagal Theory And PTSD

PTSD, or post-traumatic stress disorder, has gained considerable attention in recent years due to its occurrence among military veterans, especially those returning from the long, ongoing conflicts in the Middle East. These traumatized individuals may have experienced severe physical injuries, but in many cases, however, their injuries are psychological, resulting from their overwhelming reactions to their battlefield experiences. In earlier wars, mentally traumatized veterans were said to be suffering from shell shock, the result of seeing and feeling the consequences of war. We now recognize this condition as PTSD.

Typical symptoms of PTSD include flashbacks of the traumatic event or the inability to stop thinking about it obsessively, anxiety, depression, sleeplessness and recurring nightmares. Beyond the discomforts of experiencing PTSD, it is now known that it can lead to suicidal thoughts and suicidal behavior. In many cases, PTSD can lead to continuing deep depression and anxiety, as well as eating disorders, and substance abuse, notably drugs and alcohol.

Apart from veterans, people in all walks of life may have had terrifying, traumatic experiences, either themselves or as witnesses, that trigger PTSD, like an automobile accident, sexual or other physical assault, a serious fall at home, or loss of a loved one. Any of these extremely distressing experiences may initiate the PTSD response. Previously, victims of PTSD may have been told to shape up or get over it, but today, PTSD is a recognized, serious psychological condition requiring professional assistance to resolve. It may affect children as well as adults.

Based on the Polyvagal Theory, it is now believed by many psychologists that PTSD has its roots in the dorsal vagal response of the parasympathetic nervous system. This is the primitive freezing, or shutting down mechanism that is triggered when the person or animal faces an insurmountable or overwhelming immediate threat. When this dorsal vagal response is initiated, it can cause immobility, speechlessness, fainting and even severe shock. PTSD appears to be an ongoing form of dorsal vagal reaction.

Before reviewing the Polyvagal Theory's potential treatments for overcoming dorsal vagal-caused PTSD, an understanding of the human brain's evolution and functions is presented for perspective.

The Three-Part Brain

The human brain, with its complexity of 100 billion or so neurons and perhaps 100 trillion neural connections, is generally known to be organized into two hemispheres, the left, recognized for controlling rational, logical, organizational thoughts, and the right, associated with creative, imaginative and unstructured thinking. We also know that the functioning nervous system is comprised of the brain, spinal cord, and between them, the brainstem.

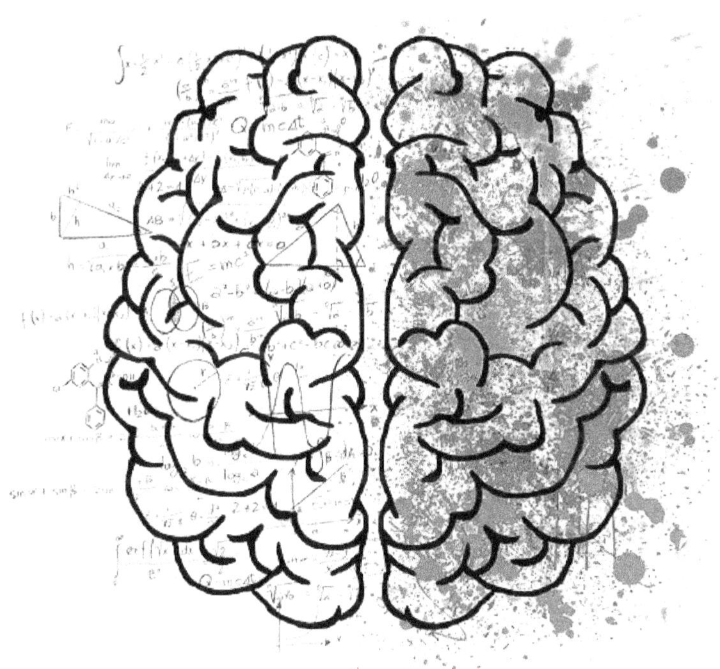

The brain is where all the conscious and unconscious action takes place, from managing our cardiovascular, respiratory and digestive functions to feelings, senses and sensations, and embracing all thought, memory and decision-making.

The spinal cord is the central cable that receives all nerve impulses from the extremities and forwards these impulses to the brain, and returns the brain's reactions to the impulses with the appropriate reaction.

The brainstem is where 10 of the 12 cranial nerves originate and extend to the organs and other key areas, including number 10, the longest, most diverse neuron, the vagus nerve.

But we know today that the evolution of the human brain has been built upon a sequential three-part structure, beginning with the earliest, most primitive part, called the reptilian brain, then continuing to evolve an early old or paleomammalian brain, and concluding with a more sophisticated new or neo-mammalian brain. This concept of a three-part evolution-driven brain structure was identified first in the 1960's by a neuroscientist, Dr. Paul MaLean, who called it the triune brain, and postulated that these three parts of the brain still struggle to coexist. Each part has specific functions to perform:

The early, reptilian brain, is responsible for basic, involuntary reflex actions, including reproduction urges, arousal to a range of stimuli and maintaining a balanced, normal state, or homeostasis. It can be considered a fundamental survival mechanism. One of its continuing characteristics is compulsiveness.

The old-mammalian, or paleomammalian brain, is positioned to surround the reptilian brain, it manages emotions, learning and memory functions. It enabled early mammals to remember and act upon favorable and unfavorable experiences, for example.

The new-mammalian, or neo-mammalian brain is responsible for conscious thought and self-awareness, and is positioned atop the two early brain parts. All of our reasoning, decision-making and rationalizations occur here.

But one may ask if we really evolved from reptiles? The concept of our brains evolving from reptiles comes as a surprise. We understand that we evolved from mammals, since we ourselves are mammals. Okay, but reptiles? Over the long course of evolution, the earliest

135

mammals evolved from, yes, reptiles, and not from the dinosaurs that became extinct 66 million years ago, or the dinosaurs that grew feathers and evolved into birds. Our reptilian ancestors were small, and obviously smarter than the large dinosaurs, which gave them an edge in natural selection. They had strong survival skills built into their small but highly functional reptilian brains, and some of these hardy reptiles evolved into small mammals. In their turn, these early mammals evolved more complex brains, the paleomammalian brain, with its added values of learning, memory and emotion. Still later, as mammals further evolved as primates, the third neo-mammalian brain component developed, giving Homo Sapiens the ability to think consciously and with increasing complexity.

The three parts of our current triune brain correspond, approximately, to the brainstem and cerebellum (reptilian), limbic brain, which includes the hippocampus, amygdala, and hypothalamus (paleomammalian) and the neocortex (neo-mammalian). Because the reptilian-originated brainstem reacts completely unconsciously and immediately for survival, historically, it tends to dominate in many situations, when the brain perceives a danger or other need for prompt action. The conflict between the purely instinctive reptilian brain and the two more advanced components is considered by some to be represented by Freud's ongoing battles between the conscious and the subconscious.

When the other dimensions and aspects of the brain are considered along with the three triune sections, the complexity of brain functioning begins to become clear. These aspects include the two-hemisphere structure, vertical networks connecting the layers and departments of the brain, and a near infinite number of interacting neurons, as well as variations in brain structure due to gender, genetic and environmental influences.

In recent times, the precise sequential evolution and functioning of the triune brain, and its exclusivity among humans have been questioned by some animal behaviorists, since complex brains have developed among non-mammal species, including certain birds. Also, new studies demonstrate that in humans, the prefrontal cortex performs complex functions that are apart from the functions of the neocortex.

Post-Traumatic Brain Reeducation

Separate from the psychological disorders associated with PTSD, there are physical brain injuries resulting in serious trauma. About 10 million people worldwide suffer traumatic brain injury (TBI) each year, and many cases are fatal, and most who survive the injury experience some degree of cognitive impairment. These trauma may occur in any number of circumstances, including vehicular accidents, sports injuries, falls inside and outside the home, acts of conflict or violence, even being struck by falling objects.

There are a range of treatments to reverse the impairment, and the type and duration of treatment depends on the type and severity of the trauma. Generally, a multidisciplinary set of treatments is required, involving the psychiatric and neurologic medical practices, as well as pharmacotherapy.

Classifying TBI as mild, moderate or severe depends on several key factors: Degree of post-traumatic consciousness, duration of the coma, if experienced by the patient, and the degree and duration of post-traumatic amnesia. Generally, TBI patients whose symptoms continue for one month or more are

138

classified as either moderate or severe, and whose full recovery make takes years, while those showing marked improvement within a few weeks are considered to be mild cases and often return to full cognitive function within two months.

There are a number of impairments to the cognitive functions following TBI. These are the most commonly treated:

- Decreased ability to concentrate

- Impaired attentiveness

- Reduced visual spatial cognizance

- Tendency to be easily distracted

- Memory lapses and impairments

- Loss of executive ability (decision-making)

- Disrupted communications skills

- Judgmental lapses and dysfunctions

Reeducation of TBI patients begins with assessments based on standardized testing protocols, including visual and auditory attentiveness, visual and verbal measurements, language comprehension and understanding, executive function (decisiveness), overall mental and intellectual function and motor function.

Post-traumatic brain reeducation is undertaken primarily through cognitive rehabilitation, which works to increase the injured person's abilities in the processing and interpretation of information, and the overall performance of mental functions. Cognitive rehabilitation is mostly effective in mild or moderate levels of TBI and with persons who have a high level of motivation to succeed in the recovery. The multidisciplinary group that collaborates on brain reeducational therapy may include doctors, speech and language specialists, physical and occupational therapists, among others. However, it is recognized that each patient's treatment will be unique, prescribed and tailored to each individual, based on the specific injuries suffered and resultant trauma.

One important approach that has wide application is attention process training (ATP), which is based on mental skills training, gradually increasing the complexity of the exercises, from simple initially, and subsequently increasing in complexity, forcing the brain to retrain itself. The exercises include selective attention, focused attentiveness, alternating attention, divided attentiveness and sustained attentiveness.

The Parasympathetic Recovery

The Polyvagal Theory links PTSD to one dimension of the parasympathetic nervous system (PNS), the early-evolved dorsal vagal freeze survival mechanism. The dorsal vagal mechanism may protect an animal by allowing it to play dead until the coast is clear, but in a human being, it can lead to inaction, inability to think or speak, or worse, passing out or fainting, shock or even cardiac arrest. With the linking of PTSD to the dorsal vagal mechanism, a previously unrecognized cause may now be open to evaluation and potentially, to alleviate the symptoms of PTSD.

Specifically, the other, more recently evolved PNS response, the calming, relaxing, socially engaging ventral vagal response may be applied to reduce the emotional and physical symptoms of PTSD. Now the methods used to achieve vagal tone and lower heart rates and breathing rates, reactivate the digestive system and induce an all-encompassing state of calm and relaxation may be applied by the individual, easily, every day. These methods, as we've discussed, include meditation, Yoga stretches and poses, and managed, deep and conscious breathing. The practice of deep, slow breathing, with forceful extension of the diaphragm to tone the vagus nerve, is applicable as part of meditation or Yoga, or simply done without other techniques.

It can also include auricular and facial massage, massage of the vagus nerve as it passes next to the right and left carotid artery in the neck, and cold facial therapy. The practice of mindfulness, or being in the moment, in which all outside thoughts are prevented from intruding, can also be beneficial, as the person concentrates on every external sound, every feeling, every awareness of things in the environment. Vocal stimulation of the vagus nerve can be done easily by singing, gargling, or reciting a mantra while performing mantra and transcendental meditation.

Another application of Polyvagal Theory to treating PTSD is for the individual to recognize that the symptoms of PTSD are biological in nature, caused by the body's primitive instincts and reflexes to protect itself, and that the body can be taught to relax, get over it, rejoin and socially engage with those who are living active, normal lifestyles. This is called somatic awareness, and it trains the individual to become aware of basic bodily functions like heart rate and breathing, and to consciously try to slow them down. The deep breathing exercises may be helpful in achieving a sense of bodily control.

The reduction or elimination of PTSD symptoms can further be achieved by practicing a series of mental exercises called attentional control, a conscious effort to recognize the cues that may trigger PTSD reactions, and gently but firmly cancel them out by acknowledging that there is no danger, nothing to fear, and all is well. This form of body awareness is called cognitive behavior therapy (CBT), and it encourages the individual to be aware that an unneeded fight or flight response is continuing and can be shut down by conscious thought, replacing disturbing thoughts and memories with relaxing, peaceful thoughts. Over time and with practice, the replacement of bad thoughts with positive ones will make the cooling down of the dorsal vagal action-orientation easier.

Reading Body Language

Body language has long been associated with a few popular positions and movements that are believed to be subconscious cues as to a person's true meaning or intentions. For example, having one's arms crossed signals a negative interest in what is being said, or a hand over one's mouth while speaking may be a sign of a lie being told. Unconsciously nodding one's head indicates agreement, a handshake suggests type of character, depending on whether it is firm or weak, and if eye contact is maintained or not. In reality, most of these body language cues are anecdotal and may have some basis, or they may not.

But Polyvagal Theory has shed a new light on body language, on multiple levels, by revealing one's interest in a social engagement, for example, or sending a signal that can trigger social engagement or other interaction in the second person, who may, in turn, respond with their own body language subconsciously. The use of facial expressions to elicit various types of responses is being used to communicate and engage with autistic children, in testimony to the effectiveness of this approach.

Do the popular body language signals really mean anything, or are they, as implied above, merely anecdotal, believed and circulated but without substantiation? A study conducted by UCLA found that only 7% of what is said is actually believed or acknowledged, based only on the words spoken. The tonality of the speaker's voice accounts for 38% of communications, leaving 50% of communications being based on body language, gestures and expressions.

Resistance to what is being said or shown is frequently shown by crossed arms and crossed legs.

A smile is not sincere when it is limited to the mouth, whereas a sincere smile engages more of the face, including crinkling the eyes.

Mirroring or imitating your own body positions is a sign that the other person is in agreement with what you are saying or proposing.

Power positions radiate a sense of command or control. A person who assumes control will tend to stand upright, extend arms and otherwise occupy more space in a room. This type of person is encouraging interaction or possibly engagement.

Eye contact is not always synonymous with engagement or interest because extended or prolonged eye contact may be forced or deliberate, suggesting the person is hiding a true intention.

Discomfort or surprise may cause raised eyebrows. Conversely, a truly interested person will not tend to raise their eyebrows when spoken to, except to acknowledge an exceptionally unusual remark.

Nodding is positive, except when it's exaggerated because too much nodding suggests discomfort with what is being said.

Tension signals stress. A furrowed brow, tightened neck muscles or a clenched jaw may be signs that what is being said is making the person uncomfortable.

Are these findings valid? Probably to some degree, but it's important to realize that the subject of body language has been widely discussed and debated for decades. As a result, many people you may be speaking with, or meet in an interview, may be consciously nodding or smiling or firmly shaking your hand, deliberately trying to make a good impression. You, in turn, might consider your own body language, and try not to send the wrong message.

The Polyvagal Theory

And Emotional Stress

Among the more profound conclusions emerging from Dr. Porges' Polyvagal Theory is the linking of the emotional and physical responses we are subject to. Emotional reactions can trigger not one but two physical responses: the well-known defensive call to action of the sympathetic nervous system, and the more primal dorsal vagal response that can freeze and immobilize a person. Physical actions, conversely, like Yoga, meditation, managed breathing and massages can tone the vagus nerve, triggering the calming, relaxing emotions of the parasympathetic nervous system (also called the ventral vagal response), and its enablement of social engagement.

Chapter 10 How To Fix Emotional Detachment

We call the state of emotional detachment, congruence.

What is congruence?

Psychological congruence is a person's ability to consistently feel and express his inner emotions with his outer world— their language of speech and body.

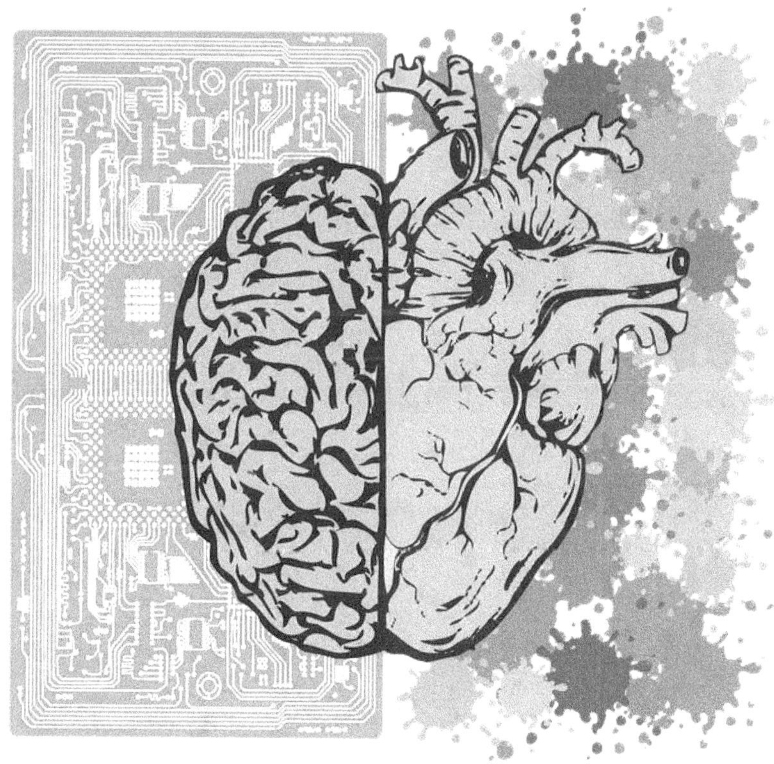

For example, when you think about something tragic, have you ever smiled? And, did you feel really upset and still keep a flat face? Have you always felt angry, but you have held her down and a headache? These are incongruous variations in terms and actions.

Incongruity happens when we have forgotten our inner world, our emotions reflected by external sensations. Many of my patients have emotions but have difficulty expressing them in words so they shake them away.

Emotions are unavoidable.

If we understand it or not, we just feel it. Common concepts include censorship, denial, coercion, and other defense mechanisms to drive them beyond our awareness for themselves. We may feel we should control our feelings, but sometimes by physical pain or sickness, they come out in one form or another.

People bury in their bodies so many of their psychological problems that they no longer feel comfortable in our bodies and we prefer to be stupid.

People push harmful feelings further from their perceptions by using narcotics, liquor and other addictions such as sex, betting, and films, or by clicking through social media indefinitely.

How do we develop incongruence?

But we do not tend to be unconnected or incongruous psychologically. When children, when we feel them, we communicate our emotions. We giggle, smile, or stick our language when we are working on a project if we are glad. We lament if we're down. We bite, shout, spit or clutch when we are angry. If we are offended, we vomit stuff out, drive them aside and condemn things!

When our feelings are mirrored and our boss understands them orally, they are well linked with our young age body responses. This is why I always encourage children to begin every punishment or high emotional moment by expressing their feelings empathically through expressions and giving sense to why they might feel that way.

Many children develop a natural, healthy ability to express feelings, which helps them work in families and relationships, over time. They know that a framework occurs to actually communicate what is happening, and that's a good thing. Sometimes it's good to block strong emotion before now!

More serious problems arise when repeated messages render our experience invalid or shameful, or when trauma keeps us away from being consistent. There may also be nobody connecting with a single person sufficiently to congruence around him.

For example, it may not be a good idea to bring out your deepest thoughts or emotions, if everyone you know would be shameful or attack you. These households often have strong drugs or alcohol, serious psychiatric illness, or a rapist.

We are meaning-making creatures. In our lives, we assign significance to events, and this is our guiding conviction and principle, especially in key childhood development periods.

These significances shape how we interact with the world. Though subconscious and involuntary, this contributes to the creation of these earlier concepts as they exist out of congruence without ourselves.

How incongruence develops:

A trauma occurs. A kid listens to a fight between his family. The child seems to be sick in the middle and distracts the parents from their struggle, thereby diminishing the struggle.

We assign meaning to it. As always, the baby refers to himself or herself as everything. They think, "If I shout if I get sick, it stops shouting."

We structure habits and actions around that belief. The person remains ill as an adaptive response to the hostility of the parent. Emotional distress and misery are thus valued when only physical pain is present.

We see patterns in our lives that reflect that belief. We respond again and again in a way that shows our confidence. Our partnerships are influenced, which further consolidates our trust in our lives. New connections to compassionate doctors are created, maybe professionals worried about medical problems, which further improve infection and are a way of responding to relaxed gaps and communication needs.

We have to either live with it or deal with it. We can not sift through the core belief until we re-examine this moment and this judgment. To incongruous men, there is an incredible possibility. The reaction to successful treatment and resulting behavioral changes can be incredible. In order to address this issue, both must find new ways to communicate with others but can not use the incongruous approach to be an efficient method.

How do we fix incongruence?

Our goal is to link up our physical body, emotion, and verbal interactions as we advance through life. From their very heart, the best public speakers seem to speak. The most important communications are to be communicated and incorporated.

We may incorporate in a number of ways the idea of reconnecting:

Art

Art helps people bypass the conceptual fields of the mind to create something pure and consistent with their internal experience. Painting, painting, playing with clay, or other art forms help us interact deep in our inner experience of things. Often we ask people to photograph themselves and create an image of their homes so they can discover new stuff and have real access.

Instead, we ask people to describe their images and to tie their shares with the congruent space of art.

True Self
154

Ginger also uses the term ' inner child,' but it is a real self, or the center of our being, that I like to represent. To live congruently from your "true self" is when you imagine what you are doing and how you are expressing yourself. This is no new idea, and my favorite author on this subject is Karen Horney's Neurosis and human development.

It can be important to discover that we have always suppressed this aspect of ourselves and to gain access to it and to benefit from it. We can find this more and more when we are around people who can give us thanks and truth as we move on.

Body scan (or interception)

Trauma patients frequently dissociate themselves from their bodies. It is easy to forget that we have bodies even in this age of engineering. Most of the time people spend unconnected by browsing the Web.

This takes us into ourselves and creates continuity as we feel the bodies and function through feelings concurrently.

If her client is having a triggering event, Ginger likes to ask questions so that she can discover the root cause of incongruity:

What is your body feeling as you talk about that?

What emotion would you name that feeling you're having?

When are you always aware of that sensation in your body? The answer of the person must be near the time of initial injury, typically in their infancy.

I like to ask as well:

As you say what are you feeling in your body?

If your body could say something what would it say?

I want to access their bodily memories and the source of their pain.

Taper off of harmful and unhelpful drugs.

The treatment for confusion is better than the source of it. It's better than that. Substances like drugs and alcohol have a profound impact on the emotions of people. In patients who treat themselves, they usually try to get rid of emotional pain symptoms.

I would like to say, "What are the things that you get out of? Dormant? Peace? Peace?"We will seek the underlying cause of where anxiety and fear and rage stems from, once we can answer the question. We will start to develop a congruence that brings peace in effect.

Individuals use illegal or prescription controlled medications to relieve psychological pain.

Instead of focusing on the signs, most doctors and therapists can be diagnosis-based. When you see a person, you will search to try to identify what is wrong to locate a drug to relieve symptoms.

When we do this as therapists, before they develop these problems, we connect to the patient's illness story rather than to who is its core.

Many patients coming to us take pills for all their various diseases 20-33 a day. When so many drugs are involved, psychotherapy can become difficult because the sensory or complete function of the brain is affected.

We also established some of these medicines if we develop a stable emotional relationship with them, and

157

then our clinicians will start building up a lot of emotions.

Through a trustful and positive connection to a psychologist, people can start to experience what is intentionally or unwittingly hidden before they start.

How can I stay congruent during tough circumstances?

It is difficult to apply to their daily lives all people have experienced during counseling. The families and friends want homeostasis — they generally want us to remain the same. "You changed," they say as if it were a bad thing.

It can be hard for our friends and family to embrace the "older us!" If we are cured or if we are congruent with ourselves, we interact more with old us.

We also found that the whole family system will change as soon as the child begins to grow.

It is not unusual to have both chronic pain and mental issues. These two things are often related, and you need to become aware of how one can affect the other.

It is natural to feel some mental anguish when in physical pain. This is because the mind and body are interconnected and influence each other greatly. An injury sustained on any part of the body, even on an area as small as a toe, can leave you feeling anxious, worried or distressed and the mind then cannot function optimally.

If you deal with chronic pain, you may eventually notice that your stress levels have become much higher and you seem to have more panic attacks, and/or you have a deepening depression.

This is often caused from the effect that chronic pain has on your mental state. At the same time, if your chronic pain is acting up and you already have anxiety or depression, those mental issues could be aggravating your pain, even though it is your mind/brain's mental response to the pain you feel.

Signs Your Pain is Causing Your Mental Issues

You may be wondering 'how will I know', if there is a link between my actual chronic pain and mental issues. The short answer is that you may never know if there is a direct link, or if you have chronic pain and a mental issue simultaneously.

However, if one did not start until the other did, there is a good chance they are connected. The good news is that if you resolve one, it might help resolve the other.

But, if you get a handle on your chronic pain, and your anxiety or depression still continues, you should seek out help for your mental issues as well.

What You Can Do About It

The best thing to do is see a professional to get both issues treated.

Physical and mental issues should be treated equally, both conditions are just as important to your overall well-being.

Don't put off getting help for mental health conditions because you don't think they are that serious, or that you can simply do it yourself. Maybe you can, but be honest, after a reasonable amount of time, if the issues persist, get some professional help!

Anxiety sufferers also remember their pain as being worse than it actually was. In studies of people undergoing dental procedures, those who had the highest levels of anxiety before the procedures not only reported higher levels of pain than control subjects, but were also the most likely to overestimate their pain three months later. Sadly, their unrealistic memories of the pain only serve to increase negative anticipation, making their next dental procedure even more painful.

Conclusion

Congratulations on making it through to the end of this journey on the vagus nerve, a scientific guide to understand how the vagus nerve determines psychological and emotional states such as anxiety, depression, migraines, back pain, and with simple exercises to improve your life.

Hopefully, it was full of information and offered tools that you need to help you achieve your goals.

The next step in your journey to understand your body and your Vagus nerve is to give stimulation techniques a shot. It is time to decide what exercises you want to try and put them into action. It is not enough to just read about all the functions of the Vagus nerve and how it can be stimulated or balanced. It is now time to apply your knowledge and change your life. And not only that, now is the time to help others learn about the Vagus nerve and how they can balance or stimulate their own. Possibly one of the most interesting outcomes of this book is that the final suggestion is to create connections with others in a genuine and wholehearted manner. And the more you build these connections the better you support their Vagus nerve stimulation, as well as your own. You can help others, ultimately help yourself, and create a more relaxed, peaceful, and balanced lifestyle. So if you are struggling with a technique outlined in this book and are unsure where to start, it is time to create these loving and kind relationships. It is time to develop deep connections with others and build a positive environment around yourself and others. This is one of the most effective methods for not only creating a great environment but also support the function of your Vagus nerve.

Thank you for reading and please take good care of your body.

People suffering from depression are often unable to take pleasure in activities they once enjoyed, and stress is part of the reason. Stress and the resulting release of glucocorticoids affect pleasure pathways in the brain, raising the threshold needed to perceive pleasure. A stressed lab rat temporarily becomes depressed, requiring stronger than normal stimulation of its pleasure pathways to elicit a sense of pleasure. Based on this research, you might guess that people taking synthetic glucocorticoids as medical treatment would experience an increased risk of depression, and you'd be right.

The effects of negative emotions on pain perception can be induced even in healthy control subjects with no chronic pain and no depressive symptoms. One study asked three groups of volunteers to read statements describing positive, neutral, or negative moods. The volunteers were then asked to try to experience their assigned mood.

As with pain and anxiety, the pain-depression relationship goes both ways; depression worsens pain and chronic pain can cause depression. The two conditions often maintain and exacerbate each other. Suffering from pain that never goes away is enough to make even the most cheerful person begin to have a negative outlook on life. Combine being in pain with the stress of missing work, the inability to do everyday activities, and feeling socially isolated, and a mood disorder seems almost inevitable.

To top it off, people in chronic pain rarely get a full, restful night of sleep. Research shows that sleep deprivation reduces your ability to control your emotions and makes you overreact to normally neutral situations. A healthy person feels grumpy when they don't sleep well for a night or two, so just imagine what months or years of inadequate sleep can do to your emotional state.